Nursing and Care Planning

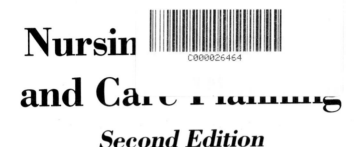

C000026464

Second Edition

Barbara J. Taptich, RN, MA

Program Director, Heart Institute
Saint Francis Medical Center
Trenton, New Jersey

Patricia W. Iyer, RN, MSN, CNA

Patricia Iyer Associates
Stockton, New Jersey

Donna Bernocchi-Losey, RN, MSN

Redwood City, California

W.B. SAUNDERS COMPANY
A Division of Harcourt Brace & Company
Philadelphia ■ London ■ Toronto ■ Montreal ■ Sydney ■ Tokyo

W.B. SAUNDERS COMPANY

A Division of Harcourt Brace & Company

The Curtis Center

Independence Square West

Philadelphia, PA 19106

Library of Congress Cataloging-in-Publication Data

Taptich, Barbara J.
  Nursing diagnosis and care planning / Barbara J. Taptich, Patricia
W. Iyer, Donna Bernocchi-Losey.—2nd ed.
    p.   cm.
  Includes bibliographical references.
  ISBN 0–7216–5196–8
  1. Nursing diagnosis. 2. Nursing care plans. I. Iyer, Patricia
W. II. Bernocchi-Losey, Donna. III. Title.
  [DNLM: 1. Nursing Diagnosis—handbooks. 2. Patient Care
Planning—handbooks. WY 39 T175n 1994]
  RT48.6.T37   1994
  616.07′5—dc20
  DNLM/DLC
                                                          93–33971

Nursing Diagnosis and Care Planning   ISBN   0–7216–5196–8

Printed in the United States of America

Last digit is the print number: 9   8   7   6   5   4   3   2

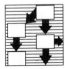

The Saunders Nursing Process Symbols depict the five steps of the nursing process through the use of shapes, arrows, and shading. In *Assessment,* the first step, the multidirectional arrows demonstrate the exploration that occurs during data collection. In *Diagnosis,* judgments are made about the assessment data, and a nursing diagnosis is derived based on these inferences. Each square in the symbol for *Planning* signifies a desired outcome of actions based on the nursing diagnosis. The directional arrows indicate that the plan is outcome-directed and client-oriented. *Intervention* involves the collaborative efforts of the nurse and client in the implementation of the nursing care plan. In this symbol, the changing tonality of the arrows connotes the client's health status as it progresses toward a high level of wellness. The arrow in the last symbol represents *Evaluation* as a flexible and ongoing process. Thus, it indicates that the nurse and client must evaluate each step of the nursing process to determine correct assessment data, an accurate nursing diagnosis, an appropriate nursing care plan, and effective nursing implementation.

About the Authors

Barbara J. Taptich, RN, MA, is the Director of the Heart Institute at Saint Francis Medical Center, Trenton, New Jersey. She has a diploma from Saint Joseph's Hospital School of Nursing, Reading, Pennsylvania, a Bachelor of Arts in Health Education and School Nursing from Glassboro State College, Glassboro, New Jersey, and a Master of Arts in Health Care Administration from Rider College, Lawrenceville, New Jersey. She was formerly the Director of Education at two community hospitals in the Trenton, New Jersey area and Instructor in Nursing Fundamentals and Critical Care Nursing at Saint Francis Medical Center School of Nursing, Trenton, New Jersey. Correspondence may be directed to the author at 20 Martin Lane, Mercerville, New Jersey 08619.

Patricia W. Iyer, RN, MSN, CNA, is president of two businesses: Patricia Iyer Associates, providing nursing consulting and educational services, and Med League Support Systems, assisting attorneys with malpractice cases. She has a diploma from Muhlenberg Hospital School of Nursing, a Bachelor of Science in Nursing, and a Master of Science in Nursing from the University of Pennsylvania. She is certified in nursing administration. Correspondence may be directed to the author at 55 Britton Road, Stockton, NJ 08559–0231.

Donna Bernocchi-Losey, RN, MSN, practices jointly with Michael L. Losey, an Internal Medicine Specialist in San Jose, California. She has a Bachelor of Science in Nursing from Seton Hall University, South Orange, New Jersey, and a Master of Arts in Nursing from New York University, New York City. She was formerly an instructor in the Department of Nursing, University of Nevada, Las Vegas, and Assistant Director of Medical/Surgical Nursing at Saint Francis Medical Center, Trenton, New Jersey. Correspondence may be directed to the author's office at 2895 The Villages Parkway, San Jose, California 95135.

Preface

Nursing Diagnosis and Care Planning, Second Edition, is designed to be used by nursing students and practicing nurses as a reference when planning nursing care.

Part I reviews current health care trends, the nursing process, and the nursing care plan. A major portion is devoted to definitions and guidelines for writing nursing diagnoses, client outcomes, and nursing interventions.

Part II presents the North American Nursing Diagnosis Association list of accepted diagnoses. The diagnoses are grouped in the classification schema known as Taxonomy I–Revised. Definitions, defining characteristics, and related factors are provided for each nursing diagnosis.

Part III consists of nursing diagnoses and client outcomes for common medical diagnoses. The medical diagnoses that were selected are representative of major categories of the Diagnostic Related Grouping (DRG) system and are those seen most frequently throughout the country.

Part IV is the differential diagnosis section, which is new to this edition. This part is designed to help the reader differentiate between commonly confused diagnoses. Definitions, defining characteristics, and related/risk factors common to each diagnosis, as well as those diagnoses which differ, are presented in an easy-to-read chart format. Case studies are included to assist the reader to discriminate between similar diagnoses.

Readers who desire more detailed information on the nursing process or nursing diagnosis should refer to the authors' complementary text:

Iyer P, Taptich B, and Bernocchi-Losey D: *Nursing Process and Nursing Diagnosis,* 2nd ed., W.B. Saunders Company, Philadelphia, 1991.

The authors wish to thank Thomas Eoyang, Editor-in-Chief, Nursing Books, W.B. Saunders Company, for his guidance, support, and patience.

Contents

Part III
Care Planning: Nursing Diagnoses and
Outcomes   185

Overview of
Care Planning

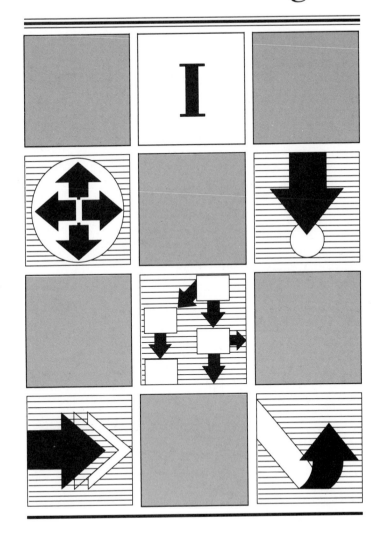

I

■ Introduction

Health Care Trends

In the 1990s a number of factors have had an impact on the health care system. As a result of these trends, nurses have experienced major changes in the delivery of nursing care. The most significant effects have resulted from the advent of prospective payment systems. Additional forces affecting nursing include the changing role of peer review organizations and the movement toward costing out nursing services.

Prospective Payment Systems

The classic example of the prospective payment system in the United States is the Diagnostic Related Grouping (DRG) system. The DRG system is a mechanism whereby health care agencies are reimbursed for services on the basis of the client's medical diagnosis. The purpose of the DRG system is to promote cost-effective health care, since it encourages prompt diagnosis, treatment, and discharge. Instead of receiving payment based on the length of the client's stay, the agency is given a fixed fee for services.

A number of factors affects the assignment of a DRG to a specific client, including age (particularly older than 70 years or younger than 18 years) and the presence or absence of surgical intervention. Other significant factors are the existence of comorbid conditions, such as diabetes and hypertension, or of complications, such as infections and emboli. The impact of prospective payment systems requires the nurse to deliver quality care to sicker clients in a compressed time frame and with fewer resources. Recently the validity of the DRG system has been questioned by many sources. The DRG system may be modified or replaced with a new system in the near future.

Peer Review Organizations

The implementation of prospective payment systems has resulted in a number of changes, particularly decreased length of stay and increased acuity. In addition to its impact on nursing services, this change precipitated the development of peer review organizations (PROs).

The purposes of PROs include the following:

1. To ensure that all health care reimbursed from federal funds is necessary
2. To ensure that care meets professional standards
3. To require that care be provided economically in an appropriate setting
4. To eliminate adverse outcomes, including premature discharges
5. To reduce unnecessary admissions and/or procedures

When evaluating the documentation of care, PRO reviewers look for answers to questions such as

1. Does the client need to be in the hospital, or could adequate care be provided in an extended-care facility or at home?
2. Do the treatments and procedures seem compatible with the client's DRG code?
3. Is the client being taught skills necessary for postdischarge care? Was discharge planned at the time of admission?
4. Are there quality-of-care issues that should have been addressed during the hospitalization?
5. If the client was readmitted to the hospital shortly after discharge, could the second admission have been prevented? Was there evidence of a premature discharge?

Costing Out Nursing Services

The issue of costing out nursing services has arisen from the prospective payment system's use of DRGs. In most hospitals the cost of nursing services is billed under room and board, but this does not take into account the varying intensity of nursing care required by patients with various medical diagnoses. "DRG systems also do not account for the range of severity of illness within a particular DRG. Federal regulations have not yet directly affected nursing reimbursement. However, there are strong indications that justifying costs for nursing service according to the patient's acuity correlated with the patient's DRG is on the horizon" (Trofino, 1986).

Additionally, since nursing costs represent a substantial portion of the total hospital budget, under- or overestimating nursing costs will place the hospital in financial jeopardy. "Documentation in the patient record of care provided in response to identified patient need and resulting patient outcome and the kind and amount of nursing time involved would allow much greater precision in cost estimates than currently available through existing nursing classification tools" (Prescott, 1986).

The end result of the changes in the health care system has been to emphasize the need for effective and efficient nursing care. This can be best accomplished by consistent utilization of the foundation of nursing: the nursing process.

The Nursing Process

The nursing process is organized into five identifiable phases: assessment, diagnosis, planning, implementation, and evaluation. Each can be described as follows.

Assessment

Assessment is the first phase of the nursing process. Its activities are focused on gathering information regarding the client, the client-family system, or the community for the purpose of identifying the client's needs, problems, concerns, or human responses. Data are collected in a systematic fashion by utilizing the interview or nursing history, physical examination, laboratory results, and other sources.

Diagnosis

During diagnosis, the data collected during assessment are critically analyzed and interpreted. Conclusions are drawn regarding the client's needs, problems, concerns, and human responses. The nursing diagnoses are identified and provide a central focus for the remainder of the phases. On the basis of the nursing diagnoses, the plan of care is designed, implemented, and evaluated. The nursing diagnoses supply an efficient method of communicating the client's problems.

Planning

In the planning phase, strategies are developed to prevent, minimize, or correct the problems identified in the nursing diagnosis. The planning phase consists of several steps:
1. Establishing priorities for the problems diagnosed
2. Setting outcomes with the client and/or family to correct, minimize, or prevent the problems
3. Writing nursing interventions that will lead to the achievement of the proposed outcomes
4. Recording nursing diagnoses, outcomes, and nursing interventions on the care plan in an organized fashion

Implementation

Implementation is the initiation and completion of the actions necessary to achieve the outcomes defined in the planning stage. It involves communication of the plan to all those participating in the client's care. The interventions can be carried out by members of the health care team, the client, or the client's family. The plan of care is used as a guide. The nurse continues to collect data regarding the client's condition and interaction with the environment. Implementation also includes recording the client's care on the proper documents. This documentation verifies that the plan of care has been carried out and can be used as a tool to evaluate the plan's effectiveness.

Evaluation

The last phase of the nursing process is evaluation. It is an ongoing process that determines the extent to which the goals of care have been achieved. The nurse assesses the progress of the client, institutes corrective measures if required, and revises the nursing care plan as needed.

This discussion has separated the nursing process into five distinct phases. In practice it is impossible to separate the phases, because they are interrelated and interdependent.

Evolution of the Care Plan

The changes in the health care delivery system have resulted in the need for rapid development of nursing diagnoses, client outcomes, and nursing interventions. The documentation of these elements has traditionally been done on the nursing care plan. The nursing care plan was originally designed as a tool for student nurses learning the nursing process. Care plans spread from the schools to a variety of settings. As nurses today struggle to deliver quality care to sicker clients in a compressed time frame with fewer resources, care planning is even more necessary.

In 1991 the Joint Commission for Accreditation of Healthcare Organizations deleted the requirement for nursing care plans. Many other regulatory agencies continue to expect nurses to prepare care plans, so they remain in existence in most settings. In addition, not all nurses agree with the Joint Commission's decision, and many maintain that nursing care plans are essential. At the same time that shifting regulations were affecting care plans, the format began changing. Practice guidelines and case management paths emerged as alternatives to traditional care plans.

Purposes

Care plans enhance the continuity of care as clients are transferred within and between agencies. Staffing patterns, which include the use of per diem, part-time, and float nurses and nurse's aides, can create situations in which staff members are unfamiliar with the client. Ultimately both staff and clients benefit from the comprehensive information found on the care plan. This information clearly communicates the client's needs and effective strategies to manage them and to encourage early and comprehensive discharge planning.

Because illness affects each person in a unique way, plans of care must be tailored to the responses and needs of each client. Rapid diagnosis of the individualized needs of the client and development of strategies to manage them are beneficial to both the client and the agency. The client's needs for personal care are met at the same time that the agency's criteria for efficient resource consumption are fulfilled.

A well-written care plan provides the blueprint for evaluation of care, because clearly defined outcomes identify the behavior that the client is expected to achieve. Consistent review of the outcomes on the care plan permits the nurse to evaluate the client's progress and to initiate necessary changes promptly.

In addition to nurses, a variety of other individuals scrutinize care plans. These include reviewers from insurance companies, PROs, and regulatory agencies; malpractice attorneys; and utilization management personnel. The information obtained is useful in validating admission, services rendered, length of stay, DRG assignment, and the delivery of quality care. A plan of care may be developed in an acute or long-term care facility, rehabilitation or home care agency, and in a variety of other settings in which nursing care is provided.

Characteristics

Regardless of the setting in which they are written, nursing care plans have certain desirable characteristics. They are as follows:
1. Written by a registered nurse
2. Initiated following the first contact with the client
3. Readily available
4. Current

Written by a Registered Nurse

The American Nurses' Association, the Joint Commission for Accreditation of Healthcare Organizations, and many nurse practice acts have addressed the development of nursing care plans. They have defined the role of the registered nurse as including responsibility for the initiation of the plan of care. On the basis of educational preparation, the registered nurse is the most qualified person to complete this function in conjunction with the client and other health care providers. The client may contribute by defining and validating outcomes and nursing interventions.

Other health care providers may be utilized in the development and implementation of the plan of care. Specific nursing activities may be delegated to other nursing personnel, such as licensed practical nurses or nursing assistants. However, the responsibility and accountability for initiating the plan of care rest with the registered nurse.

Initiated Following First Contact

The plan of care is most effective when it is initiated after the nurse's first contact with the client. Immediately after obtaining the data base, the nurse should begin to document actual, high-risk, or wellness nursing diagnoses, outcomes, and interventions. Additional interaction with the client may result in further development and refinement of the plan of care.

The nurse who obtains the data base has the most information about the client. Therefore, this nurse is most likely to be able to develop a comprehensive care plan. Occasionally, a complete data base may not be collected because of time constraints, the condition of the client, or the initiation of treatment modalities. In this situation the nurse may

1. Develop a preliminary plan based on the available information
2. Gather the absent data during subsequent contacts with the client
3. Refine the preliminary plan
4. Delegate to another registered nurse the responsibility for obtaining the absent data and refining the preliminary plan

The trend toward decreasing the length of time a client is in contact with a health care facility or service emphasizes the importance of initiating the plan on the first contact with the client. By identifying the client's needs at the time of admission, the nurse promotes efficient, coordinated care and facilitates timely discharge planning.

Readily Available

The plan of care should be readily available to all personnel involved in the care of the client. It may be placed on the client's medical record, at the bedside, or in a centralized location. Ready access to the care plan facilitates its usefulness and its value as a communication tool.

Current

Because the plan of care is the guideline for directing the client's care, it must contain current information. Therefore, it is essential that all components of the plan be updated frequently. Nursing diagnoses, outcomes, and interventions that are no longer valid are either eliminated or revised. The method of updating the plan varies with (1) the type of nursing care plan format utilized and

(2) agency policy. The continuity and individualization of the plan may be jeopardized when it is not current, and this may cause the client to lose confidence in the nurse's ability to deliver appropriate care. The plan of nursing care should be consistent with current standards of practice, which reflect the standards of professional nursing organizations and the information in nursing literature.

Format
The plan of care may be documented in several different formats, including individually developed nursing care plans, standardized care plans, teaching plans, practice guidelines, and critical paths.

Individually Developed Plans of Care
Individually prepared nursing care plans are developed both in schools of nursing and in health care facilities and agencies. They may be handwritten or developed with the assistance of a computer and then printed out. Individually (and often laboriously) developed care plans are prepared by students before they provide care on the clinical area, and they may be modified following the clinical experience. Student nursing care plans may contain components not normally found in care plans developed by graduate nurses. The extra components typically include using the plan to document the defining characteristics of the nursing diagnosis and the evaluation of the effectiveness of the plan of care. Graduate nurses usually omit documenting these components on the plan of care, because this information is found elsewhere in the clinical record.

Standardized Care Plans
In an effort to reduce the amount of effort needed to prepare individually developed care plans, standardized care plans became available in the early 1980s. These documents reflect expert opinion on the types of nursing diagnoses, outcomes, and interventions that could reasonably be expected to occur in the presence of a specific medical diagnosis. For example, the medical diagnosis of acquired immune deficiency syndrome (AIDS) may be used as the focal point for developing some of the expected nursing diagnoses seen in patients with this condition, along with examples of outcomes and interventions. Part III of this text provides some examples of nursing diagnoses and outcomes that may be present with common medical conditions.

Standardized care plans are also organized in some settings according to the nursing diagnosis. For example, a care plan could be based on the nursing diagnosis of pain, with outcomes and interventions specific to managing pain.

Most standardized care plans are designed to permit individualization by adding nursing diagnoses, time frames, or other elements to the outcomes and by modifying the interventions. Several software companies provide standardized care plan packages that can be modified according to the needs of the health care setting and to address a specific client's problems.

Teaching Plans

Teaching plans may be individually developed or standardized. Commonly, agencies will use a variety of standardized teaching plans for frequently seen learning needs, such as in clients with a myocardial infarction, mastectomy, and newly diagnosed diabetes or in clients who have just undergone labor and delivery. Teaching plans may contain nursing diagnoses and outcomes, but their primary focus is on the specific details to be taught. A section to evaluate the effectiveness of the teaching is usually included in a standardized teaching plan.

Practice Guidelines

Practice guidelines, also called protocols, define the nursing care needed for broad clinical issues such as prevention of falls or pain management. Collaborative practice guidelines identify how the medical-nursing team manages clinical concerns, such as administration of potent medications or care provided in intensive care units. Physician committees typically review newly developed collaborative practice guidelines.

Short-stay areas of a hospital, such as the labor and delivery unit, postanesthesia care unit, and the same-day surgery unit, frequently use practice guidelines. Clients who receive care in these areas often have common needs that permit the development of a practice guideline.

Nursing diagnoses, outcomes, and interventions are found in practice guidelines but are in a different format from that of the traditional three-column care plan. Additional information may include a definition of which level of nursing personnel (e.g., registered nurse, licensed practical nurse) can carry out specific components of the plan. Practice guidelines may also identify their authors and include references used to develop the plans.

Case Management or Critical Paths

The introduction of the prospective payment system has led to an intensive examination of the amount of time a client stays in a hospital. Case management originated in the outpatient setting and quickly moved into the hospitals in an effort to more effectively coordinate care resources.

A case management path, or critical path, is a preprinted standardized plan that consists of the types of activities needed to move the client through hospitalization. The path is usually based on the client's medical diagnosis, such as total hip surgery or congestive heart failure. Critical paths are interdisciplinary documents that contain the relevant activities provided by nurses, physicians, social workers, and physical and respiratory therapy personnel. A frequently used format is a calendar-like grid with components of care listed down the left side of the page and the days of stay written across the top of the page. Some critical paths incorporate nursing diagnoses and outcomes into the time frame. An increasing number of software vendors are developing programs to computerize critical paths.

When a client is unable to achieve the objectives set forth on the critical path, health care personnel attempt to analyze the reason for the variance. Variances can be due to client, system, or health care provider factors. In a separate form, the care manager, who is frequently a registered nurse, documents the reason for the variance and any follow-up action that is needed.

Components

The nursing care plan may be structured in several ways, depending on the system used in the agency. However, the nursing care plan usually consists of the following components:

1. Nursing diagnoses
2. Outcomes
3. Nursing interventions

Each of these components is examined in greater detail in the remaining pages of Part I.

■ Nursing Diagnosis

Definitions

The assessment phase of the nursing process provides the data for the nursing diagnosis. During the diagnostic phase, the nurse organizes, interprets, and validates the data obtained from the client and secondary sources. The outcome of this process is the diagnostic statement, which becomes the framework for the subsequent phases of planning, implementation, and evaluation.

A diagnosis is essentially a statement that identifies an existing undesirable state. Nurses, by virtue of their nurse practice acts, are responsible for diagnosing and treating human responses to health problems. Nursing diagnosis primarily involves areas covered by independent nursing functions, including those for which orders can be made independently, without collaboration with physicians or other health care professionals. Such functions may include (1) preventive approaches, such as education, changes of position, or observation for problems; and (2) corrective approaches, such as forcing fluids or giving treatments. This focus on independent nursing actions not only avoids duplication and overlap with other disciplines but also continues the definition and validation of the elements of nursing practice. The American Nurses' Association emphasizes the importance of nursing diagnoses in its definition of nursing: nursing is the diagnosis and treatment of human responses to actual or potential health problems (American Nurses' Association, 1980).

In 1990 the North American Nursing Diagnosis Association (NANDA) accepted the following definition of an actual nursing diagnosis: ''A nursing diagnosis is a clinical judgment about individual, family, or community responses to actual and potential health problems/life processes. Nursing diagnoses provide the basis for selection of nursing interventions to achieve outcomes for which the nurse is accountable.''

Components of the Diagnostic Statement

There are three types of nursing diagnoses: actual, high-risk, and wellness. Each is now described, and its components defined.

12

Actual Nursing Diagnosis

An actual nursing diagnostic statement consists of two parts joined by the phrase "related to." The diagnosis includes a determination of the client's problem or human response (Part I) and an identification of the etiology or related factors (Part II).

Part I: The Human Response

The first part of the diagnostic statement specifies the human response identified by the nurse during the assessment phase. This phrase provides a clear indication of what needs to change and determines the outcomes that will measure the change. Most nursing diagnoses focus on problems that the client is experiencing or is at risk of experiencing. When writing the first part of an actual diagnosis, the nurse should consider the following two areas:

1. What human response is implied by the assessment data?
2. To what degree is the human response present?

The human response can be determined by considering the list of accepted nursing diagnostic categories published by NANDA (Table 1–1). The definition and defining characteristics of each of the diagnostic categories can be found in Part II of this book.

Modifiers or qualifying phrases may also be seen in the diagnostic statement. They are utilized to identify stages or levels and are found before or after the human response. Table 1–2 lists and defines modifiers frequently used in diagnostic statements. Colons and commas may also be used to separate the various parts of the first component (see Table 1–1).

Part II: The Related Factor

The related factor (etiology) constitutes the second part of the nursing diagnostic statement. The nurse must identify the reason why a problem is occurring in order to prevent, minimize, or alleviate it. The related factor reflects the environmental, psychological, sociocultural, physiological, or spiritual elements believed to be contributing to the health problem.

Examples

Environmental	Psychological
Excessive noise	Fear of death
Noxious odors	Feelings of loneliness
Sensitivity to light	Impaired parent-infant bonding

■ Table 1—1. Alphabetical List: NANDA-Approved Diagnoses

Activity intolerance
Activity intolerance, high risk for[†]
Adjustment, impaired
Airway clearance, ineffective
Anxiety
Aspiration, high risk for[†]
Body image disturbance
Body temperature, high risk for altered[†]
Breastfeeding, effective
Breastfeeding, ineffective
Breastfeeding, interrupted*
Breathing pattern, ineffective
Cardiac output, decreased
Caregiver role strain*
Caregiver role strain, high risk for*
Communication, impaired verbal
Conflict, decisional (specify)
Conflict, parental role
Constipation
Constipation, colonic
Constipation, perceived
Coping, defensive
Coping, family: ineffective, compromised
Coping, family: ineffective, disabling
Coping, family: potential for growth
Coping, individual: ineffective
Denial, ineffective
Diarrhea
Disuse syndrome, high risk for[†]
Diversional activity deficit
Dysreflexia
Family processes, altered
Fatigue
Fear
Fluid volume deficit
Fluid volume deficit, high risk for[†]
Fluid volume excess
Gas exchange, impaired

■ **Table 1–1. Alphabetical List: NANDA-Approved Diagnoses**
Continued

Grieving, anticipatory

Grieving, dysfunctional

Growth and development, altered

Health maintenance, altered

Health-seeking behaviors (specify)

Home maintenance management, impaired

Hopelessness

Hyperthermia

Hypothermia

Incontinence, bowel

Incontinence, functional

Incontinence, reflex

Incontinence, stress

Incontinence, total

Incontinence, urge

Infant feeding pattern, ineffective*

Infection, high risk for[†]

Injury, high risk for[†]

Knowledge deficit (specify)

Mobility, impaired physical

Neurovascular dysfunction, high risk for peripheral*

Noncompliance (specify)

Nutrition, altered: high risk for more than body requirements[†]

Nutrition, altered: less than body requirements

Nutrition, altered: more than body requirements

Oral mucous membrane, altered

Pain

Pain, chronic

Parenting, altered

Parenting, altered: high risk for[†]

Personal identity disturbance

Poisoning, high risk for[†]

Post-trauma response

Powerlessness

Protection, altered

Rape-trauma syndrome

Rape-trauma syndrome: compound reaction

Table continued on following page

■ **Table 1−1. Alphabetical List: NANDA-Approved Diagnoses**
Continued

Rape-trauma syndrome: silent reaction

Relocation stress syndrome*

Role performance, altered

Self-care deficit: bathing/hygiene
                        dressing/grooming
                        feeding
                        toileting

Self-esteem, chronic low

Self-esteem disturbance

Self-esteem, situational low

Self-mutilation, high risk for*

Sensory/perceptual alterations (specify)
  (visual, auditory, kinesthetic, gustatory, tactile, olfactory)

Sexual dysfunction

Sexuality patterns, altered

Skin integrity, high risk for impaired[†]

Skin integrity, impaired

Sleep pattern disturbance

Social interaction, impaired

Social isolation

Spiritual distress

Suffocation, high risk for[†]

Swallowing, impaired

Therapeutic regimen, ineffective management of (individual)*

Thermoregulation, ineffective

Thought processes, altered

Tissue integrity, impaired

Tissue perfusion, altered (specify type)
  (cardiopulmonary, cerebral, gastrointestinal, peripheral, renal)

Trauma, high risk for[†]

Unilateral neglect

Urinary elimination, altered patterns of

Urinary retention

Ventilation, inability to sustain spontaneous*

Ventilatory weaning response, dysfunctional*

Violence, high risk for: self-directed or directed at others[†]

■ **Table 1—2. Modifiers**

Modifier	Definition	Example
Acute	Severe but of short duration	Acute pain
Altered	A change from baseline	Altered body temperature
Chronic	Lasting a long time; recurring; habitual; constant	Chronic pain
Decreased	Lessened; lesser in size, amount, or degree	Decreased cardiac output
Deficient	Inadequate in amount, quality, or degree; defective; not sufficient; incomplete	Diversional activity deficit
Depleted	Emptied wholly or partially; exhausted of	—
Disturbed	Agitated; interrupted; interfered with	Body image disturbance
Dysfunctional	Abnormal, incomplete functioning	Dysfunctional grieving
Excessive	Characterized by an amount or quantity that is greater than is necessary, desirable, or useful	Fluid volume excess
Impaired	Made worse; weakened; damaged; reduced; deteriorated	Impaired swallowing
Increased	Greater in size, amount, or degree	—
Ineffective	Not producing the desired effect	Ineffective thermoregulation
Intermittent	Stopping and starting again at intervals; periodic; cyclic	—
Potential for enhanced	For use with wellness diagnoses, *enhanced* is defined as made greater; to increase in quality; or more desired	—

Sociocultural	Physiological
Impaired ability to procure food	Swallowing difficulties
Language barrier	Sensory deficit
Lack of support systems	Abnormal fluid loss

Spiritual
Difficulty practicing religious rituals
Challenged beliefs about God
Conflict between religious beliefs and prescribed health regimen

The following are samples of diagnostic statements showing the related factor that may be associated with specific client problems.

Human Response	Related Factor
Pain	Effects of surgery
Colonic constipation	Prolonged immobility
Hypothermia	Prolonged exposure to cold
Unilateral neglect	Effects of neurological trauma
Relocation stress syndrome	Lack of support systems in new environment

The related factor helps to identify specific nursing interventions that will prevent, correct, or alleviate the problem. For example, the following diagnoses have the same human response but quite different related factors.

Human Response	Related Factor
Altered nutrition: less than body requirements	Difficulty swallowing
Altered nutrition: less than body requirements	Loss of appetite
Altered nutrition: less than body requirements	Feelings of loneliness

The nursing interventions suggested by these diagnoses also vary. Those used in the presence of swallowing difficulties might be as follows:

1. Help the client to sit upright in a 60- to 90-degree position.
2. Encourage the client to take small amounts of semisolid foods.

3. Instruct the client to place food at the back of the mouth and to think about swallowing.

If the client is experiencing loss of appetite, the following interventions may help:

1. Determine the client's food likes and dislikes.
2. Serve food in an appealing manner.
3. Provide small, frequent feedings.

For the client who does not eat because she is lonely following her husband's death, the nurse may include these interventions:

1. Encourage the client to verbalize feelings about the death of her husband.
2. Explain the hazards of continued decreased intake.
3. Arrange consultation with a psychiatric clinical specialist.
4. Provide information about support groups, such as ''Widows & Widowers'' or ''I Can Cope.''

In summary, the diagnostic statement consists of two parts linked by the words ''related to.'' The first part indicates the client's human response, and the second identifies the factors that contribute to it.

Figure 1–1 illustrates the relationship of the components of a nursing care plan, including the diagnostic statement, outcomes, and interventions.

Note that qualifying statements may be added to increase the clarity of a diagnosis (e.g., excess vs. deficit). Closely related factors may be grouped within the diagnostic statement (e.g., immobility and decreased oral intake). The nursing interventions include specific approaches for managing each factor.

Variations of the Diagnostic Statement

There are some variations in the way in which actual nursing diagnoses are written. The most common variations of the diagnostic statement are those including many related factors, the three-part diagnosis, the one-part diagnosis, and the diagnosis indicating unknown etiology.

Many Related Factors

A human response may be associated with more than one risk factor.

Example
High risk of peripheral neurovascular dysfunction can be related to effects of casting, edema, and prolonged immobility.

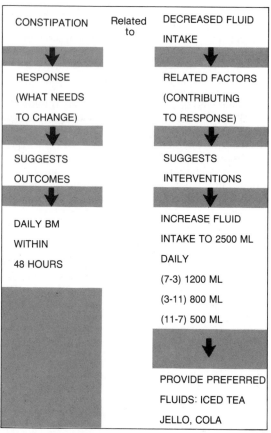

Figure 1—1. Flow chart illustrating the components of a nursing care plan, including the diagnostic statement, outcomes, and interventions. (From Iyer PW, Taptich BJ, and Bernocchi-Losey D: Nursing Process and Nursing Diagnosis, 2nd ed. Philadelphia: WB Saunders, 1991.)

At times the second part of the nursing diagnosis, or the related factor, is itself broken into two parts, connected by the words "secondary to" or the abbreviation "2°".

Example
High risk for injury related to unsteady gait secondary to side effects of medications

Three-Part Statements

Some nurses prefer to include the defining characteristics (signs and symptoms) in the nursing diagnostic statement. This is known as the PES format: *p*roblem, *e*tiology, *s*igns and *s*ymptoms. The words "as evidenced by," or the abbreviation "AEB," is placed before the signs and symptoms.

Examples
Ineffective management of therapeutic regimen (individual) related to family conflict AEB client's statement "I am not following my diet"
Ineffective infant feeding pattern related to prolonged period of being NPO AEB inability to initiate or sustain an effective suck

One-Part Statements

A few actual nursing diagnoses will be written as one-part statements without the words "related to" or an identified related factor. Examples include rape-trauma syndrome or post-trauma response, in which the etiology is obvious. In general, it is desirable to include the related factor, because it directs the nursing interventions.

Unknown Related Factor

At times the related factor will be unclear or unknown. It is acceptable to include the words "related to unknown factors" while continuing to search for the related factor.

Example
Pain related to unknown factors

High-Risk Nursing Diagnoses

Up to this point the discussion has addressed actual nursing diagnosis, the most common of the three types of nursing diagnoses. High-risk nursing diagnoses are slightly different from actual nursing diagnoses. There are two ways in which the term "high risk" is used in relation to nursing diagnoses. First, a high-risk diagnosis is now recognized as a type of nursing diagnosis. Second, the term may be used as a modifier ("high-risk") and placed in the front of a human response.

High-Risk Diagnosis as a Type of Nursing Diagnosis

In 1990 NANDA reviewed the use of the nursing diagnosis and recommended the development of a new type of nursing diagnosis; the high-risk nursing diagnosis. "A high-risk nursing diagnosis is a clinical judgment that an individual, family, or community is more vulnerable to develop the problem than others in the same or a similar situation. High-risk nursing diagnoses include risk factors that guide nursing interventions to reduce or prevent the occurrence of the problem'' (NANDA, 1990). In this definition the risk factors are behaviors, conditions, or circumstances.

Examples
High risk for infection

High risk for injury

High risk for poisoning

High risk for peripheral neurovascular dysfunction

High risk for suffocation

High risk for disuse syndrome

High risk for caregiver role strain

High risk for trauma

High risk for violence: self-directed or directed at others

High risk for self-mutilation

There are no signs, symptoms or defining characteristics for high-risk nursing diagnoses, because they represent potential, not actual, problems. The risk factor is included in the second part of the nursing diagnostic statement.

Examples
High risk for aspiration related to decreased level of consciousness

High risk for self-mutilation related to feelings of self-hatred

High-risk nursing diagnoses *may* contain risk factors that cannot be modified by nursing. For example, a client may have a high risk for poisoning related to chemical contamination of water. The nurse probably will not be able to change the presence of chemicals in the water supply but can teach the client how to avoid exposure to the water.

"High Risk" as a Modifier
In Part II of this text, definitions of the nursing diagnoses use the phrasing ''an individual experiences or is at risk for experiencing . . .'' This wording refers to the use of ''high risk'' as a modifier. In 1992 the phrase ''potential for'' was replaced with the phrase ''high risk for.'' For example, ''potential for impaired skin integrity'' became ''high risk for impaired skin integrity.'' As is true with high-risk nursing diagnoses, the term high risk as a modifier

results in risk factors being included in the second part of the nursing diagnosis.

Example
High risk for altered parenting related to hospitalization of child in ICU

Wellness Diagnoses

Wellness diagnoses focus on strengths. A wellness diagnosis is defined as a clinical judgment about an individual, family, or community in transition from a specific level of wellness to a higher level of wellness (NANDA, 1990). This type of diagnosis has one part, or the human response. It typically begins with the words "Potential for enhanced" as in "Potential for enhanced parenting" or is written as a clear statement of strengths.

Examples
Family coping, potential for growth

Health-seeking behaviors

Effective breastfeeding

Guidelines for Writing a Nursing Diagnosis

Formulation of a nursing diagnostic statement may be considered a new skill. Just like any other new skill, it takes practice. The nurse will find that with practice, the process of writing nursing diagnoses becomes easier.

One way to reduce frustration is to utilize the following guidelines when developing the diagnostic statement. These guidelines apply primarily to writing actual nursing diagnoses.

1. Write the Diagnosis in Terms of the Person's Response Rather Than Nursing Need

The first part of the diagnostic statement identifies the client's response to illness or state of health. Therapeutic or functional needs, such as "needs frequent turning" or "needs coughing and deep breathing," describe nursing interventions rather than health responses and therefore should not be included in the first part of the diagnostic statement.

Examples

Incorrect	Correct
Needs suctioning because she has many secretions	High risk for aspiration related to excessive oral secretions
Needs help with walking	Impaired physical mobility related to obesity AEB need for help when walking

2. Use "Related to" Rather Than "Due to" or "Caused by" to Connect the Two Parts of the Statement

The two parts of the diagnostic statement should always be linked together by the words "related to." This identifies a relationship between the human response and the related factor and implies that if one part of the diagnosis changes, the other part may also change. "Related to" does not necessarily mean that there is a direct cause-and-effect relationship between the two parts.

Example

Incorrect	Correct
Altered sexuality patterns caused by change in body image	Altered sexuality patterns related to change in body image

3. Write the Diagnosis in Legally Advisable Terms

A diagnostic statement such as "high risk for impaired skin integrity related to infrequent turning" is not legally advisable. This statement implies negligence or blame, which can create potential legal problems for the personnel caring for the client. This statement could be better phrased as "high risk for impaired skin integrity related to decreased mobility." The therapeutic nursing interventions would be similar in both instances, but the second statement is factual and does not imply fault.

Examples

Incorrect	Correct
High risk for trauma related to inadequately maintained skin traction	High risk for trauma related to hazards of skin traction

High risk for violence: directed at others related to inadequate supervision

High risk for violence: directed at others related to inability to cope with perceived threat to self-esteem

4. Write the Diagnosis Without Value Judgments

Nursing diagnoses should be based on objective and subjective data collected and validated in cooperation with the client or significant other. The behavior of the client should not be judged by the nurse's personal values and standards. The use of words such as "inadequate," "poor," and "unhealthy" frequently implies value judgments.

Examples

Incorrect	Correct
Altered parenting related to poor bonding with child	Altered parenting related to prolonged separation from child
Caregiver role strain related to irresponsible behavior of caregiver	Caregiver role strain related to caregiver's marginal coping patterns

5. Avoid Reversing the Parts

Remember that the first part of the diagnostic statement reflects the human response and defines outcomes. The second part of the statement identifies the related factors and suggests nursing interventions. Reversing the parts may result in unclear communication about the client's problem and its related factor. This would make it difficult to write appropriate outcomes and nursing interventions.

Examples

Incorrect	Correct
Confinement to home related to impaired social interaction	Impaired social interaction related to confinement to home
Increased caloric intake related to altered nutrition: more than body requirements	Altered nutrition: more than body requirements related to increased caloric intake

6. Avoid Including Signs and Symptoms of Illness in the First Part of the Statement

The first part of the diagnostic statement is derived from a cluster of signs and symptoms observed by the nurse during the assessment of the client. An isolated sign or symptom is not a nursing diagnosis, but it may provide clues to help identify the problem. Inaccurate diagnoses may occur if the nurse focuses on an isolated sign or symptom rather than on the entire clinical picture. Although some of the human responses on the NANDA list look like symptoms, such as pain, fatigue, or constipation, they actually represent a cluster of signs and symptoms. For example, a person in acute pain may be moaning, clutching the body part, and having increased cardiac and respiratory rates.

Example

Incorrect	Correct
Withdrawn behavior related to inability to engage in satisfying personal relationships	Social isolation related to inability to engage in satisfying personal relationships

7. Be Sure That the Two Parts of the Diagnosis Do Not Mean the Same Thing

In some instances diagnostic statements are written in which the two parts say the same thing. Examine this statement: "impaired adjustment related to inability to adjust." Both parts of the statement have the same meaning. The diagnostic statement should be written as "impaired adjustment related to effects of moving to new school."

Examples

Incorrect	Correct
Stress incontinence related to inability to control urine	Stress incontinence related to impaired muscle tone AEB loss of urine when standing
Dysfunctional ventilatory weaning response related to inability to adjust to lowered levels of mechanical ventilation	Dysfunctional ventilatory weaning response related to uncontrolled pain

8. Express the Problem and Related Factors in Terms That Can Be Changed

Keep in mind that the diagnostic statement identifies actual or high-risk client responses. These responses and the factors that contribute to their presence should be changeable by intervention within the realm of nursing practice. One of the most common errors nurses make when writing nursing diagnoses is to include a related factor that cannot be changed by nursing practice. For example, nurses cannot change the fact that a client has had surgery or is dying from cancer. However, we can help the client to manage the effects of medical diagnoses and life processes.

Examples

Incorrect	Correct
Knowledge deficit (pregnancy)	Knowledge deficit (prenatal diet)
Ineffective airway clearance related to chronic obstructive pulmonary disease	Ineffective airway clearance related to retained secretions AEB ineffective cough

9. State the Diagnosis Clearly and Concisely

Clear, concise diagnostic statements facilitate communication and allow the nurse to concentrate on the factors contributing to the existence of a specific problem. In writing clear diagnostic statements, be sure that the related factor can be easily associated with the first part of the diagnosis.

Example

Incorrect	Correct
Fatigue related to dizziness	High risk for trauma related to dizziness

Diagnostic statements should be as concise as possible, since wordy statements tend to obscure the focus of the nursing diagnosis.

Example

Incorrect	Correct
Ineffective individual coping related to belief that she caused onset of premature labor by lifting paint can on day of delivery	Ineffective individual coping related to feelings of guilt

Before committing the diagnosis to paper, it is helpful to verify its accuracy. This can be accomplished by asking the following questions:

1. Do you have a comprehensive data base that reflects both history and physical assessment?
2. Can you identify a pattern?
3. Does the definition of the human response you have selected seem consistent with the pattern you have identified?
4. Does the assessment data match the defining characteristics of the nursing diagnosis you have selected? (See Part II of this book.)
5. Does (do) the related factor(s) you have identified correspond to those associated with the human response?
6. Does the nursing diagnosis identify a response that can be managed by nursing intervention?
7. When appropriate, can the diagnosis be verified with the client by describing the problem and asking if the client agrees?

After you have verified the accuracy of the diagnostic statement, include it on the plan of care.

The next step in the care planning process is the development of patient-centered outcomes.

Correctly Stated Nursing Diagnoses

Chronic pain related to effects of back injury
Impaired adjustment related to inadequate support systems
Impaired swallowing related to limited awareness
Altered sexuality patterns related to fear of pregnancy
Inability to sustain spontaneous ventilation related to respiratory muscle fatigue AEB dyspnea
Altered thought processes related to sleep deprivation
High risk for infection related to effects of chemotherapy

■ Outcomes

Purposes

Nursing diagnostic statements primarily identify actual or high risk for responses that are considered to be problems for the client. This implies that alternative responses are required or preferred. Development of outcomes is an element of the planning process. It also provides a blueprint for the evaluation component. Concise, measurable outcomes that are also reasonable allow the nurse and client to evaluate the client's progress toward the desired outcome as well as the effectiveness of nursing interventions.

Outcomes also help to define specific behaviors that demonstrate that the problem has been corrected, minimized, or prevented. The outcomes identified below demonstrate alternative behaviors.

Nursing Diagnosis	Outcome
Altered nutrition: less than body requirements related to chewing difficulties (broken dentures)	Consumes 1800 calories of pureed and liquid foods each 24 hours
High risk for impaired skin integrity related to irritating stomal drainage	Skin around stoma free of redness, excoriation throughout hospitalization

Guidelines for Writing Outcomes

The rules that guide the formulation of outcomes are based on the premise that outcomes should be easily understandable. A clearly written outcome enhances communication and continuity of care. Nursing personnel who use the plan of care should be able to read an outcome and understand what it means. The following rules serve as guidelines for writing understandable outcomes.

1. Outcomes Should Be Related to the Human Response

Outcomes should reflect the first half of the diagnostic statement by identifying alternative healthful responses that are desirable for the client. At times nurses may write outcomes that are correctly worded but do not correspond to the first part of the diagnostic statement.

Example

Nursing Diagnosis: Altered nutrition: less than body requirements related to decreased appetite

Incorrect Outcome	Correct Outcome
Throughout hospitalization: no evidence of skin breakdown over bony prominences	Weight loss does not exceed 3 lb during hospitalization

Note that the corrected outcome is more closely related to the client's nutritional status. If the outcome regarding skin breakdown is a valid concern, this indicates the need to initiate a second diagnosis, "high risk for impaired skin integrity related to altered nutritional status." The outcome for this diagnosis might be "No evidence of skin breakdown throughout hospitalization."

2. Outcomes Should Be Client-Centered

Outcomes are written to focus on the behavior of the client. The outcome should address what the client will do, and when and to what extent it will be accomplished. Nursing activities and nursing goals should not be the focus of the outcome.

Example

Nursing Diagnosis: Relocation stress syndrome related to effects of transfer to long-term care facility AEB mental confusion

Incorrect Outcome	Correct Outcome
Prevent increased confusion (nursing goal)	Return to baseline mental functioning within 2 weeks

3. Outcomes Should Be Clear and Concise

Ambiguous or abstract wording should be avoided, since it may confuse rather than help the staff caring for a client. Use simple terms and standard terminology. The outcome should have as few words as possible yet still be clear. Long, involved outcomes can frequently be stated in fewer words.

Example

Nursing Diagnosis: Knowledge deficit (surgical experience)

Incorrect Outcome	Correct Outcome
The client will discuss expectations of this hospitalization and previous hospital admissions and will discuss impending surgery with a basic knowledge of hospital routine	Prior to surgery, discusses expectations of hospitalization and surgery

Eliminate the words "the client will" at the beginning of outcomes. It should be obvious from the way the outcome is stated that it is referring to the behaviors the client will exhibit. Outcomes that address the behavior of the client *and* family or significant other arise when these individuals are expected to demonstrate certain knowledge or skills as a result of teaching.

Example

Nursing diagnosis: High risk for injury related to daughter's lack of knowledge of morphine pump functioning

Outcome: Prior to discharge daughter accurately administers morphine drip by pump

4. Outcomes Should Be Observable and Measurable

Previously it was stated that the outcome should address what the client will do, and when and to what extent it will be accomplished. Observable and measurable outcomes include the "what" and "to what extent."

Example

Nursing Diagnosis: Ineffective management of therapeutic regimen related to lack of knowledge of techniques to avoid infection

Incorrect Outcome	Correct Outcome
Understands the importance of avoiding infection	By 10/23 demonstrates improved management of therapeutic regimen by performing return demonstration of dressing changes using clean technique

It is impossible to evaluate someone's understanding of a concept. The client's knowledge of techniques to avoid infection can be measured by the statements of the client and by observing how the client changes the dressing. When outcomes are measurable, observations can be made to determine whether they have been achieved.

Example

Nursing Diagnosis: Fluid volume deficit related to persistent nausea and vomiting

Incorrect Outcome	Correct Outcome
Drinks adequate amounts of fluid	Drinks 3000 ml in 24 hours

5. Outcomes Should Be Time-Limited

The time for achievement of the outcome should be stated. Examples of time-limited statements include the phrases "by the time of discharge," "throughout hospitalization," "by the end of the teaching session," and "within 48 hours." These suggest the time frame for evaluating the achievement of each outcome.

Example

Nursing Diagnosis: Sleep pattern disturbance related to unfamiliar environment

Incorrect Outcome	Correct Outcome
States she can sleep	Within 2 days states she is sleeping for at least 4 hours at a time

6. Outcomes Should Be Realistic

The outcomes should be achievable with the resources of the client, nursing staff, and agency. The client's readiness to achieve the outcomes will be affected by many factors, including finances, level of intelligence, and emotional and physical condition.

Examples

The Ideal	The Reality
Measures blood glucose level accurately with glucometer	The client cannot afford to purchase a glucometer
Spends 4 hours a day in a gerichair	There are two gerichairs on a 30-bed unit

7. Outcomes Should Be Determined by the Client and Nurse Together

During the initial assessment, the nurse begins involving the client in the planning of care. In the interview the nurse learns about what the client sees as the primary health problem. This leads to the formulation of nursing diagnoses. The client and nurse discuss the outcomes and plan of care to validate them. In this discussion they communicate their expectations. Together they have an opportunity to modify any unrealistic outcomes. The inclusion of the client as an active participant in the plan of care helps ensure the achievement of the outcomes.

Example
Sophie Lean is a 68-year-old diabetic who is admitted with diabetic retinopathy and gangrene of the left foot. During the interview Sophie asks the nurse to review the care of her feet. The nurse says, "By the time you leave the hospital, we will review how to wash and dry your feet, the signs of an infection, and what to do if you find an infection. How does this sound?" Sophie says, "Yes, that's what I want."

During this conversation the nurse has set outcomes and validated them with Sophie. By the time of discharge, the client will

1. Demonstrate proper foot care
2. Describe signs of infection
3. State the course of action to follow if infection occurs.

Correctly Stated Outcomes

Following teaching session, describes three activities that reduce anginal episodes

After nutrition class, names the four basic food groups for school nurse

By the time of discharge, transfers safely from bed to wheelchair

Temperature within normal limits 2 hours after administration of acetaminophen

Verbalizes acceptance of impending death

By the end of home teaching session, utilizes sterile technique to inject self with insulin

No evidence of accident or injury in home after correction of safety hazards

Weight loss of at least 3 lb in 2 weeks

Participates in social activities at least twice per week

Eats all meals in dining room within 1 week

■ Nursing Interventions

Following the development of nursing diagnoses and client-centered outcomes, the nurse develops nursing interventions.

Nursing interventions are specific approaches designed to assist the client to achieve outcomes. They are based on (1) the related factor in the nursing diagnostic statement, (2) the information obtained during the assessment interview, (3) the nurse's subsequent interactions with the client and family, (4) the feasibility of successfully implementing the intervention, (5) the acceptability of the intervention to the client, and (6) the capabilities of the nurse.

Nursing interventions define (1) how the nurse will assist the client to achieve the proposed outcomes and (2) the interdependent and independent nursing functions that will be required to eliminate the factors contributing to the problem.

Components of Nursing Interventions

Nursing interventions provide the health care team with a blueprint for reaching the established outcomes and resolving the unhealthful responses. A set of nursing interventions should be written to accomplish each outcome. In order to be effective, the nursing interventions must be written as clearly and concisely as possible.

Types of Nursing Interventions

Nursing interventions focus on the activities required to promote, maintain, or restore the client's health. They may be categorized as interdependent or independent.

Physician-Initiated Orders

Medical orders, or physician-initiated orders, are usually transcribed onto a Kardex or computer work sheet. These orders may be integrated into the plan of care as appropriate. Some authors refer to these orders as "dependent orders" or "collaborative actions."

Example
Demerol 100 mg IM prn q4h

Interdependent Interventions

Interdependent nursing interventions describe the activities that the nurse carries out in cooperation with other health care team members. The interventions may involve collaboration with social workers, dietitians, therapists, technicians, and physicians.

Example

Douglas Bleakley is a client who is in renal failure. The medical order states "restrict fluids to 600 ml by mouth plus 720 ml 5% dextrose in 0.45 sodium chloride solution IV every 24 hours." To define how this will be achieved, the nurse and dietitian calculate the amount of fluid Douglas may receive each shift. The nursing interventions are as follows:

1. Run IV fluids via pump @ 30 ml/hour
2. Restrict PO fluid intake:
   Day shift—315 ml (240 ml on tray, 75 ml for medication)
   Evening shift—195 ml (120 ml on tray, 75 ml for medication)
   Night shift—100 ml (for medication)

Independent Interventions

Independent nursing interventions are the activities that may be performed by the nurse without a direct physician's order. The types of activities that nurses may order independently are defined by nursing diagnoses. They are the responses that nurses are licensed to treat by virtue of their education and experience and are the primary focus of nursing diagnoses.

Example

Constance Barrett is an 82-year-old woman who fell and broke her hip. She says to the nurse, "I am going to have to watch myself when I go home. I don't want to hurt myself again." The rehabilitation nurse writes the following interventions:

"Assist the client to identify potential hazards at home."

"Notify the client's son of concerns and seek his involvement in correcting hazards."

"Encourage the client to request home hazard survey by the visiting nurse prior to discharge."

Guidelines for Writing Nursing Interventions

1. Nursing Interventions Should Be Dated and Signed

The date identifies the initiation of specific nursing interventions and allows the nurse to evaluate the client's progress toward achieving the outcomes. The signature emphasizes the nurse's legal and personal accountability.

2. Nursing Interventions Should Include Precise Action Verbs and List Specific Activities to Achieve the Desired Outcomes

All nursing interventions should clearly communicate the expected activities. Action verbs are useful in defining specific interventions, since verbs that are not precise create confusion for the caregiver. Interventions may begin with verbs such as "assess," "monitor," "instruct," "report," and so on.

Incorrect	Correct
Encourage progressive activity	Encourage client to stay out of bed in chair for 2 hours at a time

3. Nursing Interventions Should Define Who, What, Where, When, How and How Often Other Identified Activities Will Take Place

The following are suggestions for how to write clearly defined interventions:

a. Specify who will complete the interventions if other than the nurse implementing the plan of care (e.g., client, family, consultant)

Example
Instruct family on use of glucagon to treat hypoglycemia

b. List the specific activities to be implemented in order to accomplish the identified outcomes

Example
Teach client to use abdominal breathing techniques when experiencing stress

c. Define where, when, and how often the activities will take place

Example
Ambulate from bed to bathroom after meals twice daily

d. Describe how the activity should be implemented.

Example
Nursing Diagnosis—High risk for trauma related to dizziness and weakness

Outcome—Throughout hospitalization no evidence of injury
Interventions—
    (1) encourage use of railings when in bathroom and hall,
    (2) keep room free of obstacles,
    (3) keep siderails up at all times,
    (4) keep items within reach on bedside stand,
    (5) instruct client to call for help before getting out of bed

4. Nursing Interventions Should Be Consistent with the Plan of Care

The nursing interventions should not be in conflict with the thera-peutic approaches of other members of the health team. Confusion and frustration result when nurses and other professionals are work-ing at cross-purposes. It is important that members of various disciplines communicate their goals and define approaches to achieve those goals.

Example
Reinforce dietitian's teaching by monitoring client's food selection from daily menu

5. Nursing Interventions Should Be Based on Scientific Principles

The nursing interventions prescribed for an individual client should evolve from sound nursing judgment. A scientific rationale supports the nurse's decisions and forms the foundation for nursing action. This rationale is developed from the nurse's knowledge base, which includes natural and behavioral sciences and the humanities. Care plans developed by student nurses may include the rationale, but this is not commonly documented on plans of care written by graduate nurses.

Examples

Nursing Intervention	Scientific Principle
Encourage parents to identify hazards in the home	Toddlers are at high risk for injuries and falls in the home
Teach client to rotate insulin injection sites	Repeated use of the same site may cause fibrosis, scarring, and decreased insulin absorption

6. Nursing Interventions Should Be Individualized to the Client

One purpose of nursing interventions is to communicate how one client's care differs from that of another with a similar nursing or medical diagnosis. When developing nursing interventions, the nurse chooses approaches that address the client's specific physical and emotional needs. In the following example, note that although the nursing diagnosis is the same for both clients, the nursing interventions are individualized.

Examples

Nursing Diagnosis: High risk for impaired skin integrity related to immobility

Dona (Age 17)	Betsey (Age 84)
1. Apply foam mattress to bed	1. Apply air mattress to bed
2. Encourage client to use trapeze to change position	2. Assist client to change position q2h (see turning schedule); include prone position at least once per shift

---

Correctly Stated Nursing Interventions

Monitor vital signs q2h (even).
Observe IV site for redness, swelling, and edema q shift.
Turn q2h (odd) according to turning schedule.
Assess skin for redness or breakdown q2h when turning.
Instruct client's husband in dressing change procedure on 10/30.
Observe client's husband performing dressing change on 10/31.
Wake client at 6 A.M. and assist to bathroom.
Discuss side effects of antihypertensive medications, and instruct client to see nurse practitioner if symptomatic.
Instruct child's teacher to observe for signs/symptoms of petit mal seizures.
Assist client to identify support systems available within the community.

7. Nursing Interventions Should Include Modifications of Standard Therapy

Nurses utilize a variety of standard procedures to implement patient care. It is not necessary to incorporate the entire procedure in the plan of care. Occasionally, however, modifications must be made, and these should be specific in the nursing interventions.

Example

A modification of Hickman catheter care might read: "Perform Hickman catheter care three times weekly—Monday, Wednesday, and Friday. Do not use Betadine—client is allergic."

Bibliography

American Nurses' Association: Nursing: A Social Policy Statement. Kansas City, MO: American Nurses' Association, 1980.

Edelstein J: A study of nursing documentation. Nursing Management 21(11):40, 1990.

Greve P: Documentation: Every word counts. RN July:55, 1992.

Hays J: Voices in the record. Image 21(4):200, 1989.

Iyer P, and Camp N: Nursing Documentation: A Nursing Process Approach. St. Louis: Mosby–Year Book, 1991.

Iyer P: New trends in charting. Nursing 91 1:48, 1991.

Kerr S: A comparison of four nursing documentation systems. Journal of Nursing Staff Development January/February:26, 1992.

Miller D: Complying with Joint Commission nursing standards: Practical documentation tools. Journal of Healthcare Quality 14:24, 1992.

NANDA News. Nursing Diagnosis 1(3):124, 1990.

Neubauer M: Careful charting—your best defense. RN: November:77, 1990.

Prescott P: DRG prospective reimbursement: The nursing intensity factor. Nursing Management 17(1):4346, 1986.

Qamar S: An integrated nursing care plan. Nursing Management 21(5):96T, 1990.

Smith M, and Dugan J: Nursing model encourages care planning. Journal of Continuing Education in Nursing 21(1):32, 1990.

Trofino J: A reality based system for pricing nursing service. Nursing Management 17(1):1924, 1986.

Approved Nursing Diagnoses

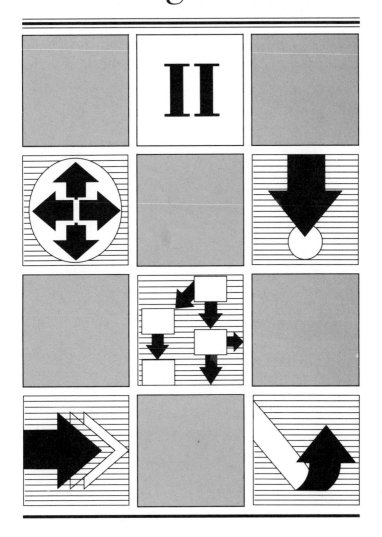

II

The currently accepted North American Nursing Diagnosis Association (NANDA) diagnoses are organized in a classification known as Taxonomy I. NANDA adopted this grouping to facilitate the organization of nursing diagnoses. Nurses can expect that this ordering may change, since Taxonomy I, as the first step in organizing this information, will be tested, refined, revised, and expanded.

Taxonomy I is organized to reflect the patterns of human responses, which are listed and defined below:

1. *Exchanging*—A human response pattern involving mutual giving and receiving
2. *Communicating*—A human response pattern involving sending messages
3. *Relating*—A human response pattern involving established bonds
4. *Valuing*—A human response pattern involving the assigning of relative worth
5. *Choosing*—A human response pattern involving the selection of alternatives
6. *Moving*—A human response pattern involving activity
7. *Perceiving*—A human response pattern involving the reception of information
8. *Knowing*—A human response pattern involving meaning associated with information
9. *Feeling*—A human response pattern involving the subjective awareness of information

Table 2–1 illustrates the groupings of accepted diagnoses, which have been placed under each human response pattern.

This part of the book is organized according to Taxonomy I, including the revisions made at the 1992 NANDA conference. In addition to providing the currently accepted NANDA diagnoses, this section includes the definition, defining characteristics, and related factors for each of the diagnoses. Readers can refer to this section for assistance in formulating correctly stated nursing diagnoses—an important component of nursing care planning. For ease of use, an alphabetized list of diagnoses has been provided on pages 48–50 and inside the front and back covers of the book.

■ **Table 2—1. Patterns of Human Responses**

Pattern 1: Exchanging

1.1.2.1	Altered nutrition: more than body requirements
1.1.2.2	Altered nutrition: less than body requirements
1.1.2.3	Altered nutrition: high risk for more than body requirements[†]
1.2.1.1	High risk for infection[†]
1.2.2.1	High risk for altered body temperature[†]
1.2.2.2	Hypothermia
1.2.2.3	Hyperthermia
1.2.2.4	Ineffective thermoregulation
1.2.3.1	Dysreflexia
1.3.1.1	Constipation
1.3.1.1.1	Perceived constipation
1.3.1.1.2	Colonic constipation
1.3.1.2	Diarrhea
1.3.1.3	Bowel incontinence
1.3.2	Altered patterns of urinary elimination
1.3.2.1.1	Stress incontinence
1.3.2.1.2	Reflex incontinence
1.3.2.1.3	Urge incontinence
1.3.2.1.4	Functional incontinence
1.3.2.1.5	Total incontinence
1.3.2.2	Urinary retention
1.4.1.1	Altered (specify type) tissue perfusion (renal, cerebral, cardiopulmonary, gastrointestinal, peripheral)
1.4.1.2.1	Fluid volume excess
1.4.1.2.2.1	Fluid volume deficit
1.4.1.2.2.2	High risk for fluid volume deficit[†]
1.4.2.1	Decreased cardiac output
1.5.1.1	Impaired gas exchange
1.5.1.2	Ineffective airway clearance
1.5.1.3	Ineffective breathing pattern
1.5.1.3.1	Inability to sustain spontaneous ventilation*

■ **Table 2—1. Patterns of Human Responses** *Continued*

1.5.1.3.2	Dysfunctional venilatory weaning response*
1.6.1	High risk for injury†
1.6.1.1	High risk for suffocation†
1.6.1.2	High risk for poisoning†
1.6.1.3	High risk for trauma†
1.6.1.4	High risk for aspiration†
1.6.1.5	High risk for disuse syndrome†
1.6.2	Altered protection
1.6.2.1	Impaired tissue integrity
1.6.2.1.1	Altered oral mucous membrane
1.6.2.1.2.1	Impaired skin intregrity
1.6.2.1.2.2	High risk for impaired skin integrity†

Pattern 2: Communicating

2.1.1.1	Impaired verbal communication

Pattern 3: Relating

3.1.1	Impaired social interaction
3.1.2	Social isolation
3.2.1	Altered role performance
3.2.1.1.1	Altered parenting
3.2.1.1.2	High risk for altered parenting†
3.2.1.2.1	Sexual dysfunction
3.2.2	Altered family processes
3.2.2.1	Caregiver role strain*
3.2.2.2	High risk for caregiver role strain*
3.2.3.1	Parental role conflict
3.3	Altered sexuality patterns

Pattern 4: Valuing

4.1.1	Spiritual distress (distress of the human spirit)

Pattern 5: Choosing

5.1.1.1	Ineffective individual coping
5.1.1.1.1	Impaired adjustment

Table continued on following page

■ **Table 2−1. Patterns of Human Responses** *Continued*

5.1.1.1.2	Defensive coping
5.1.1.1.3	Ineffective denial
5.1.2.1.1	Ineffective family coping: disabling
5.1.2.1.2	Ineffective family coping: compromised
5.1.2.2	Family coping: potential for growth
5.2.1	Ineffective management of therapeutic regimen (individual)*
5.2.1.1	Noncompliance (specify)
5.3.1.1	Decisional conflict (specify)
5.4	Health-seeking behaviors (specify)

Pattern 6: Moving

6.1.1.1	Impaired physical mobility
6.1.1.1.1	High risk for peripheral neurovascular dysfunction*
6.1.1.2	Activity intolerance
6.1.1.2.1	Fatigue
6.1.1.3	High risk for activity intolerance[†]
6.2.1	Sleep pattern disturbance
6.3.1.1	Diversional activity deficit
6.4.1.1	Impaired home maintenance management
6.4.2	Altered health maintenance
6.5.1	Feeding self-care deficit
6.5.1.1	Impaired swallowing
6.5.1.2	Ineffective breastfeeding
6.5.1.2.1	Interrupted breastfeeding*
6.5.1.3	Effective breastfeeding
6.5.1.4	Ineffective infant feeding pattern*
6.5.2	Bathing/hygiene self-care deficit
6.5.3	Dressing/grooming self-care deficit
6.5.4	Toileting self-care deficit
6.6	Altered growth and development
6.7	Relocation stress syndrome*

■ **Table 2–1. Patterns of Human Responses** *Continued*

Pattern 7: Perceiving

7.1.1	Body image disturbance
7.1.2	Self-esteem disturbance
7.1.2.1	Chronic low self-esteem
7.1.2.2	Situational low self-esteem
7.1.3	Personal identity disturbance
7.2	Sensory/perceptual alterations (specify) (visual, auditory, kinesthetic, gustatory, tactile, olfactory)
7.2.1.1	Unilateral neglect
7.3.1	Hopelessness
7.3.2	Powerlessness

Pattern 8: Knowing

8.1.1	Knowledge deficit (specify)
8.3	Altered thought processes

Pattern 9: Feeling

9.1.1	Pain
9.1.1.1	Chronic pain
9.2.1.1	Dysfunctional grieving
9.2.1.2	Anticipatory grieving
9.2.2	High risk for violence: self-directed or directed at others[†]
9.2.2.1	High risk for self-mutilation*
9.2.3	Post-trauma response
9.2.3.1	Rape-trauma syndrome
9.2.3.1.1	Rape-trauma syndome: compound reaction
9.2.3.1.2	Rape-trauma syndrome: silent reaction
9.3.1	Anxiety
9.3.2	Fear

* New diagnostic categories approved 1992.
† Categories with modified label terminology.

Alphabetical Index of Nanda-Approved Diagnoses

Activity intolerence
Activity intolerance, high risk for[†]
Adjustment, impaired
Airway clearance, ineffective
Anxiety
Aspiration, high risk for[†]
Body image disturbance
Body temperature, high risk for altered[†]
Breastfeeding, effective
Breastfeeding, ineffective
Breastfeeding, interrupted[*]
Breathing pattern, ineffective
Cardiac output, decreased
Caregiver role strain[*]
Caregiver role strain, high risk for[*]
Communication, impaired verbal
Conflict, decisional (specify)
Conflict, parental role
Constipation
Constipation, colonic
Constipation, perceived
Coping, defensive
Coping, family: ineffective, compromised
Coping, family: ineffective, disabling
Coping, family: potential for growth
Coping, individual: ineffective
Denial, ineffective
Diarrhea
Disuse syndrome, high risk for[†]
Diversional activity deficit
Dysreflexia
Family processes, altered
Fatigue
Fear
Fluid volume deficit
Fluid volume deficit, high risk for[†]
Fluid volume excess
Gas exchange, impaired
Grieving, anticipatory
Grieving, dysfunctional
Growth and development, altered
Health maintenance, altered
Health-seeking behaviors (specify)

Home maintenance management, impaired
Hopelessness
Hyperthermia
Hypothermia
Incontinence, bowel
Incontinence, functional
Incontinence, reflex
Incontinence, stress
Incontinence, total
Incontinence, urge
Infant feeding pattern, ineffective*
Infection, high risk for[†]
Injury, high risk for[†]
Knowledge deficit (specify)
Mobility, impaired physical
Neurovascular dysfunction, high risk for peripheral*
Noncompliance (specify)
Nutrition, altered: high risk for more than body requirements[†]
Nutrition, altered: less than body requirements
Nutrition, altered: more than body requirements
Oral mucous membrane, altered
Pain
Pain, chronic
Parenting, altered
Parenting, altered: high risk for[†]
Personal identity disturbance
Poisoning, high risk for[†]
Post-trauma response
Powerlessness
Protection, altered
Rape-trauma syndrome
Rape-trauma syndrome: compound reaction
Rape-trauma syndrome: silent reaction
Relocation stress syndrome*
Role performance, altered
Self-care deficit: bathing/hygiene
                  dressing/grooming
                  feeding
                  toileting
Self-esteem, chronic low
Self-esteem disturbance
Self-esteem, situational low
Self-mutilation, high risk for*
Sensory/perceptual alterations (specify)
   (visual, auditory, kinesthetic, gustatory, tactile, olfactory)
Sexual dysfunction
Sexuality patterns, altered

Skin integrity, high risk for impaired[†]
Skin integrity, impaired
Sleep pattern disturbance
Social interaction, impaired
Social isolation
Spiritual distress
Suffocation, high risk for[†]
Swallowing, impaired
Therapeutic regimen (individual), ineffective management of[*]
Thermoregulation, ineffective
Thought processes, altered
Tissue integrity, impaired
Tissue perfusion, altered (specify type)
    (cardiopulmonary, cerebral, gastrointestinal, peripheral, renal)
Trauma, high risk for [†]
Unilateral neglect
Urinary elimination, altered patterns of
Urinary retention
Ventilation, inability to sustain spontaneous[*]
Ventilatory weaning response, dysfunctional[*]
Violence, high risk for: self-directed or directed at others[†]

[*] New diagnoses, 1992.
[†] Modified label terminology, 1992.

Exchanging
A human response pattern involving mutual giving and receiving

 Diagnosis: *Altered Nutrition: More than Body Requirements*

Definition: The state in which the individual consumes more than adequate nutritional intake in relation to metabolic demands

Defining Characteristics
Weight 10%–20% over ideal for height and frame
Triceps skin fold greater than 15 mm in men, 25 mm in women
Measured food consumption exceeds American Diabetic Association recommendations for activity level, age, sex
Reported or observed dysfunctional eating patterns
    Pairing food with other activities
    Concentrating food intake at end of day
    Eating in response to external cues, such as time of day or social situation
    Eating in response to internal cues other than hunger, such as anxiety or stress
Sedentary activity level

Related Factors
Lack of
    Physical exercise
    Social support for weight loss
    Knowledge regarding nutritional needs
Decreased activity pattern
Imbalance between activity level and caloric intake
Eating in response to stress or emotional trauma
Eating as a comfort measure/substitute gratification
Learned eating behaviors
Decreased metabolic need
Weight gain during pregnancy over current recommendations
Effects of drug therapy (appetite-stimulating)
Ethnic and cultural values
Negative body image
Perceived lack of control
Decreased self-esteem
Feelings of anxiety, depression, guilt, boredom, frustration

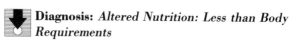 **Diagnosis:** *Altered Nutrition: Less than Body Requirements*

Definition: The state in which the individual consumes insufficient nutritional intake in relation to metabolic demands

Defining Characteristics
> Loss of weight with adequate food intake
> Body weight 20% or more less than ideal for height and frame
> Reported altered taste sensation
> Satiety immediately after ingesting food
> Abdominal pain with or without pathology
> Sore, inflamed buccal cavity
> Capillary fragility
> Abdominal cramping
> Diarrhea and/or steatorrhea
> Hyperactive bowel sounds
> Pale conjunctival and mucous membranes
> Poor muscle tone or skin turgor
> Excessive hair loss
> Decreased serum albumin or total protein
> Decreased serum transferrin or iron-binding capacity
> Metabolic demands in excess of intake
> Anemia
> Lack of interest in food
> Perceived inability to ingest food
> Reported or evidence of lack of food
> Aversion to eating
> Reported inadequate food intake less than recommended daily allowance (RDA)
> Weakness of muscles required for swallowing or mastication
> Lack of information, misinformation
> Misconceptions

Related Factors
> Inability to ingest or digest food or absorb nutrients owing to biological, psychological, or economic factors; for example:
> > Impaired absorption
> > Alteration in taste or smell
> > Dysphagia
> > Dyspnea
> > Stomatitis
> > Nausea and vomiting
> > Fatigue
> > Inability to chew

Decreased appetite
Decreased salivation
Effects of hyperanabolic or catabolic states: cancer, burns, infections
Decreased level of consciousness
Stress
Effects of aging—decreased sense of taste
Knowledge deficit
Inadequate finances

High-Risk Diagnosis: *Altered Nutrition: High Risk for More than Body Requirements*

Definition: The condition in which the individual is at risk of experiencing excessive nutritional intake in relation to metabolic demands

Risk Factors

> Reported or observed obesity in one or both parents
>
> Rapid transition across growth percentiles in infants or children
>
> Reported use of solid food as major food source before 5 months of age
>
> Observed use of food as reward or comfort measure
>
> Reported or observed higher baseline weight at beginning of each pregnancy
>
> Dysfunctional eating patterns
>
>> Pairing food with other activities
>>
>> Concentrating food intake at end of day
>>
>> Eating in response to external cues such as time of day, social situation
>>
>> Eating in response to internal cues other than hunger, such as anxiety, stress

High-Risk Diagnosis: *High Risk for Infection*

Definition: The state in which an individual is at increased risk for being invaded by pathogenic organisms

Risk Factors
- Inadequate primary defenses
    - Broken skin
    - Traumatized tissue
    - Decreased ciliary action
    - Stasis of body fluids
    - Change in pH of secretions
    - Altered peristalsis
- Inadequate secondary defenses
    - Decreased hemoglobin
    - Leukopenia
    - Suppressed inflammatory response
- Tissue destruction and increased environmental exposure
- Effects of
    - Chronic disease
    - Immunosuppression
    - Inadequate acquired immunity
    - Invasive treatments/procedures
    - Malnutrition
    - Pharmaceutical agents
    - Trauma
- Rupture of amniotic membranes
- Insufficient knowledge to avoid exposure to pathogens

High-Risk Diagnosis: *High Risk for Altered Body Temperature*

Definition: The state in which the individual is at risk for failure to maintain body temperature within normal range

Risk Factors

Dehydration
Inactivity or vigorous activity
Altered metabolic rate
Medications causing vasoconstriction/vasodilation
Sedation
Illness or trauma affecting temperature regulation
Extremes of age
Extremes of weight
Exposure to cold/cool or warm/hot environments
Inappropriate clothing for environmental temperature

Diagnosis: *Hypothermia*

Definition: The state in which an individual's body temperature is reduced to below the normal range

Defining Characteristics
>Major
>>Reduction in body temperature below the normal range
>>Shivering (mild)
>>Cool skin
>>Pallor (moderate)
>Minor
>>Slow capillary refill
>>Tachycardia
>>Cyanotic nail beds
>>Hypertension
>>Piloerection
>>Verbalization of feeling cold

Related Factors
>Effects of
>>Aging
>>Exposure to cool or cold environment
>>Illness or trauma
>>Damage to hypothalamus
>>Inability or decreased ability to shiver
>>Medications causing vasodilation
>Malnutrition
>Inadequate clothing
>Consumption of alcohol
>Evaporation from skin in cool environment
>Decreased metabolic rate
>Inactivity

Diagnosis: *Hyperthermia*

Definition: The state in which the individual is at risk because the body temperature is elevated above the individual's normal range

Defining Characteristics
    Major
        Increase in body temperature above normal range
    Minor
        Skin flushed or warm to the touch
        Increased respiratory rate
        Tachycardia
        Seizures/convulsions
        Shivering
        Weakness, faintness
        Perspiration
        Verbal reports of feeling hot

Related Factors
    Exposure to hot environment
    Increased metabolic rate
    Effects of
        Medications/anesthesia
        Illness or trauma involving temperature regulation
        Aging
        Obesity
    Dehydration
    Inability or decreased ability to perspire
    Vigorous activity
    Inappropriate clothing
    Inability to regulate environmental temperature
        No air conditioning
        Isolette temperature for infants

Diagnosis: *Ineffective Thermoregulation*

Definition: The state in which the individual's temperature fluctuates between hypothermia and hyperthermia

Defining characteristics
Fluctuation in body temperature above and below the normal range

See also major and minor characteristics present in hypothermia and hyperthermia

Related Factors
Effects of
Trauma or illness
Immaturity
Confusion
Aging
Fluctuating environmental temperature
Sedation
Medications causing vasoconstriction or vasodilation
Extremes of age
Extremes of weight
Inappropriate clothing for environmental temperature

Diagnosis: *Dysreflexia*

Definition: The state in which an individual with a spinal cord injury at T7 or above experiences a life-threatening uninhibited sympathetic response of the nervous system to a noxious stimulus

Defining Characteristics

Major: Individual with spinal cord injury (T7 or above) with:

Paroxysmal hypertension (sudden periodic elevated blood pressure where systolic pressure is over 140 mmHg and diastolic pressure is above 90 mmHg)

Bradycardia or tachycardia (pulse rate of less than 60 or over 100 beats/min)

Diaphoresis (above the injury)

Red splotches on skin (above the injury)

Pallor (below the injury)

Headache (a diffuse pain in different portions of the head and not confined to any nerve distribution on the head)

Minor

Chilling

Conjunctival congestion

Horner's syndrome (constriction of the pupil, partial ptosis of the eyelid, enophthalmos, and sometimes loss of sweating over the affected side of the face)

Paresthesia

Pilomotor reflex (gooseflesh formation when skin is cooled)

Blurred vision

Chest pain

Metallic taste in mouth

Nasal congestion

Related Factors

Bladder distention

Bowel distention

Constipation

Skin irritation

Lack of client/caregiver knowledge

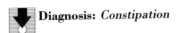 **Diagnosis:** *Constipation*

Definition: The state in which the individual experiences a change in normal bowel habits characterized by a decrease in frequency and/or passage of hard, dry stools

Defining Characteristics
Decreased activity level
Frequency less than usual pattern
Hard, formed stools
Palpable mass
Straining at stool
Palpable hard stool on rectal examination
Less than usual amount of stool
Decreased bowel sounds
Gas pain and flatulence
Abdominal or back pain
Reported feeling of abdominal or rectal fullness/pressure
Reported use of laxatives
Impaired appetite
Headache
Nausea
Irritability
Interference with daily living

Related Factors
Less than adequate
    Dietary intake
    Fiber intake
    Fluid intake
Gastrointestinal lesions
Pain/discomfort on defecation
Effects of
    Aging
    Diagnostic procedures
    Medication
    Neuromuscular/musculoskeletal impairment
    Pregnancy
    Presence of anatomical obstruction
    Stress or anxiety
Weak abdominal musculature
Immobility or less than adequate physical activity
Chronic use of laxatives and enemas
Personal habits
Ignoring urge to defecate
Fear of rectal or cardiac pain

Diagnosis: *Perceived Constipation*

Definition: The state in which an individual makes a self-diagnosis of constipation and ensures a daily bowel movement through abuse of laxatives, enemas, and suppositories

Defining Characteristics
> Major
>> Expectation of a daily bowel movement with the resulting overuse of laxatives, enemas, or suppositories
>> Expected passage of stool at the same time every day

Related Factors
> Cultural/family health beliefs
> Faulty appraisal
> Impaired thought processes

Diagnosis: *Colonic Constipation*

Definition: The state in which an individual's pattern of elimination is characterized by hard, dry stool that results from a delay in passage of food residue

Defining Characteristics
> Major
>> Decreased frequency
>> Hard, dry stool
>> Straining at stool
>> Painful defecation
>> Abdominal distention
>> Palpable mass
> Minor
>> Rectal pressure
>> Headache
>> Appetite impairment
>> Abdominal pain

Related Factors
> Less than adequate
>> Fluid intake
>> Dietary intake
>> Fiber intake
>> Physical activity
> Immobility
> Lack of privacy
> Emotional disturbances
> Chronic use of medication and enemas
> Stress
> Change in daily routine
> Metabolic problems
>> Hypothyroidism
>> Hypocalcemia
>> Hypokalemia

Diagnosis: *Diarrhea*

Definition: The state in which the individual experiences a change in normal bowel habits characterized by the frequent passage of fluid, loose or unformed stools

Defining Characteristics
    Abdominal pain
    Anorexia
    Change in color or odor of stool
    Chills
    Cramping
    Fatigue
    Fever
    Increased frequency of bowel sounds
    Increased frequency of stool
    Irritated anal area
    Loose, liquid stools
    Malaise
    Mucoid stool
    Muscle weakness
    Thirst
    Urgency
    Weight loss

Related Factors
    Allergies
    Effects of
        Medications
        Radiation
        Surgical intervention
    Infectious process
    Inflammatory process
    Malabsorption syndrome
    Nutritional disorders
    Stress and anxiety
    Dietary alterations
        Food intolerances
        High cellulose foods
        Increased caffeine consumption
        Hyperosmolar tube feeding
    Excessive use of laxatives
    Ingestion of contaminated water or food

Diagnosis: *Bowel Incontinence*

Definition: The state in which an individual experiences a change in normal bowel habits characterized by involuntary passage of stool

Defining Characteristics

Involuntary passage of stool
Lack of awareness of need to defecate
Lack of awareness of passage of stool
Rectal oozing of stool
Urgency

Related Factors

Diarrhea
Impaction
Effects of
    Cognitive impairment
    Medications
    Neuromuscular impairment
    Perceptual impairment
Large stool volume
Depression
Severe anxiety
Physical or psychological barriers that prevent access to an
    acceptable toileting area
Excessive use of laxatives

Diagnosis: *Altered Patterns of Urinary Elimination* .

Definition: The state in which an individual experiences a disturbance in urine elimination

Defining Characteristics
- Distended bladder
- Dysuria
- Frequency
- Hesitancy
- Incontinence
- Increase or decrease in total urine voided in 24 hours, in proportion to intake
- Nocturia
- Retention
- Urgency

Related Factors
- Anatomical obstruction
- Constipation/fecal impaction
- Dehydration
- Fatigue
- Obesity
- Mechanical trauma
- Pain/spasm in bladder or abdomen
- Urinary tract infection
- Decreased attention to bladder cues
  - Depression
  - Sedation
  - Confusion
- Fear
- Inability to express needs
- Stress
- Change in environment
- Effects of
  - Aging
  - Immobility
  - Indwelling catheter
  - Medications
  - Pregnancy
  - Sensorimotor impairment
  - Surgery
- Lack of privacy
- Prolonged bedrest

Diagnosis: *Stress Incontinence*

Definition: The state in which an individual experiences a loss of urine of less than 50 ml occurring with increased abdominal pressure

Defining Characteristics
    Major
        Dribbling associated with increased abdominal pressure/ exercise
    Minor
        Frequency (more often than every 2 hours)
        Loss of urine in standing position
        Urgency

Related Factors
    Degenerative changes in pelvic muscles and structural supports associated with increased age
    Effects of
        Pregnancy
        High abdominal pressure
        Obesity
    Incompetent bladder outlet
    Overdistention between voidings
    Weak pelvic muscles and structural supports

Diagnosis: *Reflex Incontinence*

Definition: The state in which an individual experiences an involuntary passage of urine occurring at predictable intervals when a specific bladder volume is reached

Defining Characteristics
> Lack of
>> Awareness of being incontinent
>> Awareness of bladder filling
>> Urge to void or feelings of fullness
> Somewhat predictable voiding pattern
> Uninhibited bladder contractions/spasm at regular intervals
> Voiding in large amounts

Related Factors
> Effects of neurological impairment
>> Cerebral loss
>> Interruption of spinal nerve impulse above the level of S3

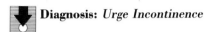 **Diagnosis:** *Urge Incontinence*

Definition: The state in which an individual experiences involuntary passage of urine occurring soon after a strong sense of urgency to void

Defining Characteristics
Major
  Bladder contracture/spasm
  Frequency (voiding more often than every 2 hours)
  Urinary urgency
Minor
  Nocturia (more than twice per night)
  Voiding in large amounts (more than 550 ml)
  Voiding in small amounts (less than 100 ml)
  Inability to reach toilet in time

Related Factors
Bladder infection/irritation
Changes in urine concentration
Decreased bladder capacity associated with
  Abdominal surgeries
  History of pelvic inflammatory disease
  Indwelling catheter
Overdistention of bladder
Diuretic therapy
Ingestion of
  Alcohol
  Caffeine
  Increased fluids

Diagnosis: *Functional Incontinence*

Definition: The state in which an individual experiences involuntary and unpredictable passage of urine

Defining Characteristics
Urge to void or bladder contractions sufficiently strong to result in loss of urine before reaching an appropriate site or receptacle
Unpredictable voiding pattern
Unrecognized signals of bladder fullness

Related Factors
Effects of
Cognitive deficits
Motor deficits
Sensory deficits
Altered environment

Diagnosis: *Total Incontinence*

Definition: The state in which an individual experiences a continuous and unpredictable passage of urine

Defining Characteristics
> Constant flow of urine occurs at unpredictable times without distention
> Incontinence refractory to therapy
> Lack of awareness of
>> Perineal or bladder filling
>> Incontinence
> Nocturia
> Uninhibited bladder contractions/spasms
> Unsuccessful incontinence refractor treatments

Related Factors
> Effects of
>> Fistulas secondary to trauma
>> Independent contraction of detrusor reflex due to surgery
>> Neurological dysfunction causing triggering of micturition at unpredictable times
>> Neuromuscular trauma related to surgical procedures
>> Neuropathy preventing transmission of reflex indicating bladder fullness
>> Trauma or disease affecting spinal cord/nerves

Diagnosis: *Urinary Retention*

Definition: The state in which an individual experiences incomplete emptying of the bladder

Defining Characteristics
>Bladder distention
>Diminished force of urinary stream
>Dribbling
>Dysuria
>Hesitancy
>High residual urine (more than 150 ml, or 20% of voided urine)
>Nocturia
>Overflow incontinence
>Sensation of bladder fullness
>Small, frequent voiding or absence of urine output

Related Factors
>Effects of
>>Anxiety (fear of postoperative pain)
>>Diminished or absent sensory and/or motor impulses
>>Inhibition of reflex arc
>>Medications
>>>Anesthetics
>>>Opiates
>>>Psychotropics
>>High urethral pressure caused by weak detrusor
>>Strong sphincter
>>Urethral blockage associated with
>>>Fecal impaction
>>>Postpartum edema
>>>Prostate hypertrophy
>>>Surgical swelling

Diagnosis: *Altered (Specify Type) Tissue Perfusion: Renal, Cardiopulmonary, Cerebral, Gastrointestinal, Peripheral*

Definition: The state in which an individual experiences a decrease in nutrition and oxygenation at the cellular level due to a deficit in capillary blood supply

Defining Characteristics
    Renal
        Diminished urine output
        Edema
    Cardiopulmonary
        Chest pain (relieved by rest)
        Increased heart rate
        Increased respiratory rate
        Shortness of breath
    Cerebral
        Alteration in thought processes
        Blurred vision
        Changes in level of consciousness
        Confusion
        Restlessness
        Syncope/vertigo
    Gastrointestinal
        Constipation
        Nausea and vomiting
        Pain
    Peripheral
        Altered sensory or motor function
        Burning
        Changes in hair pattern
        Claudication
        Coolness of skin
        Diminished pulse quality
        Edema
        Erythema
        Extremity pain
        Flushing
        Inflammation
        Pallor
        Positive Homans' sign
        Shining skin
        Slow growth, brittle nails
        Tissue necrosis (gangrene)

Text continued on following page

Diagnosis: *Altered (Specify Type) Tissue Perfusion:*
Renal, Cardiopulmonary, Cerebral,
   Gastrointestinal, Peripheral (Continued)

Trophic skin changes
Ulcerated skin/poorly healing areas

Related Factors
Exchange problems
Hypervolemia
Hypovolemia
Interruption of flow
   Arterial
   Venous

Diagnosis: *Fluid Volume Excess*

Definition: The state in which an individual experiences increased fluid retention and edema

Defining Characteristics
> Abnormal breath sounds; rales (crackles)
> Anasarca
> Azotemia
> Changes in
>> Blood pressure
>> Central venous pressure
>> Electrolytes
>> Hemoglobin and hematocrit
>> Mental status
>> Pulmonary artery pressure
>> Respiratory pattern
>> Specific gravity
>
> Edema
> Effusion
> Intake greater than output
> Jugular vein distention
> Muscular twitching/weakness
> Nausea and/or vomiting
> Oliguria
> Positive hepatojugular reflex
> Pulmonary congestion on chest x-ray
> Shortness of breath, orthopnea
> S3 heart sound
> Weight gain
> Restlessness and anxiety

Related Factors
> Compromised regulatory mechanisms
>> Aldosterone
>> Antidiuretic hormone
>> Renin-angiotensin
>
> Effects of
>> Age extremes
>> Medications
>> Pregnancy
>
> Excessive fluid or sodium intake
> Low protein intake

Diagnosis: *Fluid Volume Deficit*

Definition: The state in which an individual experiences vascular, cellular, or intracellular dehydration

Defining Characteristics
> Changes in
>> Urine output
>> Urine concentration
>> Serum sodium
>
> Sudden weight loss or gain
> Decreased venous filling
> Hemoconcentration
> Hypotension
> Thirst
> Increased
>> Pulse rate
>> Body temperature
>
> Decreased
>> Skin turgor
>> Pulse volume/pressure
>
> Change in mental state
> Dry skin
> Dry mucous membranes
> Weakness

Related Factors
> Active fluid volume loss
> Failure of regulatory mechanisms

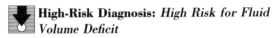 **High-Risk Diagnosis:** *High Risk for Fluid Volume Deficit*

Definition: The state in which an individual is at risk of experiencing vascular, cellular, or intracellular dehydration

Risk Factors

 Extremes of age

 Extremes of weight

 Excessive losses through normal routes, e.g., diarrhea

 Losses through abnormal routes, e.g., indwelling tubes

 Deviations affecting access to or intake or absorption of fluids, e.g., physical immobility

 Factors influencing fluid needs, e.g., hypermetabolic state

 Knowledge deficit related to fluid volume

 Effects of medications, e.g., diuretics

Diagnosis: *Decreased Cardiac Output*

Definition: A state in which the blood pumped by an individual's heart is sufficiently reduced that it is inadequate to meet the needs of the body's tissues

Defining Characteristics
>Abnormal heart sounds
Altered blood gases
Anorexia
Changes in
>>Blood pressure
Color of skin or mucous membranes
Mental status
>Cold, clammy skin
Cough
Decreased peripheral pulses
Dyspnea
Dysrhythmias, electrocardiographic changes
Edema of trunk, sacrum, or extremities
Fatigue
Frothy sputum
Gallop rhythm
Jugular vein distention
Oliguria
Orthopnea
Rales
Restlessness
Shortness of breath
Sudden weight gain
Syncope
Tachycardia
Variations in hemodynamic readings
Vertigo
Weakness

Related Factors
>Reduction in stroke volume as a result of
>>Electrical malfunction
>>>Alteration in conduction
Alteration in rate
Alteration in rhythm

Mechanical malfunction
    Alteration in afterload
    Alteration in inotropic changes in heart
    Alteration in preload
Structural problems secondary to congenital abnormal-
   ities, trauma

Diagnosis: *Impaired Gas Exchange*

Definition: The state in which an individual experiences a decreased passage of oxygen and/or carbon dioxide between the alveoli and the vascular system

Defining Characteristics
 Clubbing of fingers
 Confusion
 Cyanosis
 Fatigue and lethargy
 Hypercapnea
 Hypoxia
 Inability to move secretions
 Irritability
 Restlessness
 Somnolence
 Tachycardia
 Use of accessory muscles

Related Factors
 Ventilation-perfusion imbalance
 Altered
  Blood flow
  Oxygen-carrying capacity of blood
  Oxygen supply
 Alveolar-capillary membrane changes
 Aspiration of foreign matter
 Decreased surfactant production
 Effects of
  Anesthesia
  Medications (narcotics, sedatives, tranquilizers)
 Hypo-/hyperventilation
 Inhalation of toxic fumes or substances

Diagnosis: *Ineffective Airway Clearance*

Definition: The state in which an individual is unable to clear secretions or obstructions from the respiratory tract to maintain airway patency

Defining Characteristics
>Absent or adventitious breath sounds
>Air hunger
>Change in respiratory rate or depth
>Cough, effective or ineffective, with or without sputum
>Cyanosis
>Diaphoresis
>Dyspnea
>Fever
>Restlessness
>Stridor
>Substernal, intercostal retraction
>Tachycardia
>Tachypnea
>Anxiety

Related Factors
>Decreased energy, fatigue
>Effects of
>>Anesthesia
>>Infection
>>Medication (narcotics, sedatives, tranquilizers)
>>Perceptual/cognitive impairment
>>Presence of artificial airway
>>Trauma
>Inability to cough effectively
>Tracheobronchial secretions or obstruction
>Aspiration of foreign matter
>Environmental pollutants
>Inhalation of toxic fumes or substances

Diagnosis: *Ineffective Breathing Pattern*

Definition: The state in which an individual's inhalation and/or exhalation pattern does not enable adequate pulmonary inflation or emptying

Defining Characteristics
>Abnormal blood gases
Altered chest excursion
Assumption of three-point position
Cough
Cyanosis
Dyspnea
Fremitus
Increased anteroposterior diameter
Nasal flaring
Pursed-lip breathing and prolonged expiratory phase
Respiratory rate, depth changes
Shortness of breath
Tachypnea
Use of accessory muscles

Related Factors
>Decreased
>>Energy
Lung expansion
>Effects of
>>Anesthesia
Cognitive/perceptual impairment
Medication (narcotics, sedatives, tranquilizers)
Neuromuscular/musculoskeletal impairment
Obesity
>Fatigue
Immobility, inactivity
Inflammatory process
Pain, discomfort
Tracheobronchial obstruction
Anxiety

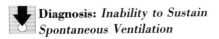 **Diagnosis:** *Inability to Sustain Spontaneous Ventilation*

Definition: A state in which the response pattern of decreased energy reserves results in an individual's ability to maintain breathing adequate to support life

Defining Characteristics
> Major
>> Dyspnea
>> Increased metabolic rate
> Minor
>> Increased restlessness
>> Apprehension
>> Increased use of accessory muscles
>> Decreased tidal volume
>> Increased heart rate
>> Decreased pO_2
>> Increased pCO_2
>> Decreased cooperation
>> Decreased SaO_2

Related Factors
> Metabolic factors
> Respiratory muscle fatigue

Diagnosis: *Dysfunctional Ventilatory Weaning Response (DVWR)*

Definition: A state in which a patient cannot adjust to lowered levels of mechanical ventilator support, which interrupts and prolongs the weaning process

Defining Characteristics
> Mild DVWR
>> Major
>>> Responds to lowered levels of mechanical ventilator support with
>>> Restlessness
>>> Slightly increased respiratory response
>> Minor
>>> Responds to lowered levels of mechanical ventilator support with
>>> Expressed feelings of increased need for oxygen; breathing discomfort, fatigue, warmth
>>> Queries about possible machine malfunction
>>> Increased concentration on breathing
> Moderate DVWR
>> Major
>>> Responds to lowered levels of mechanical ventilator support with
>>> Slight increase from baseline blood pressure < 20 mmHg
>>> Slight increase from baseline heart rate < 20 beats/min
>>> Baseline increase in respiratory rate < 5 breaths/min
>> Minor
>>> Hypervigilence to activities
>>> Inability to respond to coaching
>>> Inability to cooperate
>>> Apprehension
>>> Diaphoresis
>>> Eye widening, "wide-eyed look"
>>> Decreased air entry on auscultation
>>> Color changes; pale, slight cyanosis
>>> Slight respiratory accessory muscle use
> Severe DVWR
>> Major
>>> Responds to lowered levels of mechanical ventilator support with
>>> Agitation

Deterioration in arterial blood gases from current
baseline
Increase from baseline blood pressure > 20 mmHg
Increase from baseline heart rate > 20 beats/min
Respiratory rate increases significantly from
baseline

Minor

Profuse diaphoresis
Full respiratory accessory muscle use
Shallow, gasping breaths
Paradoxical abdominal breathing
Discoordinated breathing with the ventilator
Decreased level of consciousness
Adventitious breath sounds, audible airway secre-
tions
Cyanosis

Related Factors

Physical

Ineffective airway clearance
Sleep pattern disturbance
Inadequate nutrition
Uncontrolled pain or discomfort

Psychosocial

Knowledge deficit of the weaning process, patient role
Patient-perceived inefficiency about the ability to wean
Decreased motivation
Decreased self-esteem
Anxiety: moderate, severe
Fear
Hopelessness
Powerlessness
Insufficient trust in the nurse

Situational

Uncontrolled episodic energy demands or problems
Inappropriate pacing of diminished ventilator support
Inadequate social support
Adverse environment (noisy, active environment, nega-
tive events in the room, low nurse-to-patient ratio,
extended nurse absence from the bedside)
History of ventilator dependence > 1 week
History of multiple unsuccessful weaning attempts

High-Risk Diagnosis: *High Risk for Injury*

Definition: The state in which an individual is at risk of injury as a result of environmental conditions interacting with the individual's adaptive and defensive resources

Risk Factors
> Internal
>> Biochemical
>> Regulatory dysfunction (sensory, integrative, effector dysfunction; tissue hypoxia)
>> Malnutrition
>> Immune/autoimmune
>> Abnormal blood profile (leukocytosis/leukopenia, altered clotting factors, thrombocytopenia, sickle cell, thalassemia, decreased hemoglobin)
>> Physical (broken skin, altered mobility)
>> Developmental age (physiological, psychosocial)
>> Psychological (affective, orientation)
> External
>> Biological (immunization level of community, microorganism)
>> Chemical (pollutants, poisons, drugs, pharmaceutical agents, alcohol, caffeine, nicotine, preservatives, cosmetics and dyes)
>> Nutrients (vitamins, food types)
>> Physical (design, structure and arrangement of community, building, and/or equipment)
>> Mode of transport/transportation
>> People/provider (nosocomial agents, staffing patterns; cognitive, affective, and psychomotor factors)

High-Risk Diagnosis: *High Risk for Suffocation*

Definition: The state in which an individual has accentuated risk of accidental suffocation (inadequate air available for inhalation)

Risk Factors
> *Internal (Individual)*
>> Disease or injury process
>> Lack of
>>> Safety education
>>> Safety precautions
>> Reduced
>>> Motor abilities
>>> Olfactory sensation
>> Cognitive or emotional difficulties
> *External (Environmental)*
>> Children
>>> Inserting small objects into mouth or nose
>>> Left unattended in tubs or pools
>>> Playing with plastic bags, balloons
>> Discarded or unused refrigerators, freezers with doors not removed
>> Household gas leaks
>> Immobile client incorrectly positioned on abdomen
>> Low-strung clothesline
>> Pacifier hung around infant's neck
>> Person who eats large mouthfuls of food
>> Pillows placed
>>> In an infant's crib
>>> Incorrectly under the head of client with a compromised airway
>> Propped bottle placed in an infant's crib
>> Smoking in bed
>> Use of fuel-burning heaters not vented to outside
>> Vehicle engine running in closed garage
>> Ventilator connectors improperly monitored

High-Risk Diagnosis: *High Risk for Poisoning*

Definition: The state in which an individual has accentuated risk for accidental exposure to or ingestion of drugs or dangerous products in doses sufficient to cause poisoning

Risk Factors
> *Internal (Individual)*
>> Reduced vision
>> Cognitive or emotional difficulties
>> Inadequate drug education
>>> Combination of drugs/alcohol
>>> Consumption of outdated drugs
>>> Use of drugs prescribed for others
>> Insufficient finances
>> Lack of safety, proper precautions
>
> *External (Environmental)*
>> Availability of illicit drugs contaminated by poisonous additives
>> Chemical contamination of food, water
>> Dangerous products, medicines placed or stored within the reach of children or confused persons
>> Flaking, peeling paint or plaster in presence of young children
>> Large supplies of drugs in home
>> Paint, lacquer in poorly ventilated areas or without effective protection
>> Poisons stored in food containers
>> Presence of
>>> Atmospheric pollutants
>>> Poisonous vegetation
>> Unprotected contact with heavy metals or chemicals
>> Unsafe work environment

High-Risk Diagnosis: *High Risk for Trauma*

Definition: The state in which an individual has accentuated risk of accidental tissue injury associated with internal or external factors

Risk Factors
    Internal (Individual)
        Balancing difficulties
        Confusion
        Fatigue
        Hypotension
            Orthostatic
            Postural
        Pain
        Poor vision
        Reduced
            Hand-eye coordination
            Large, small muscle coordination
            Mobility of arms, legs
            Temperature, tactile sensation
        Side effects of medications
        Visual, hearing impairment
        Weakness
        History of
            Previous trauma
            Substance abuse
        Insufficient finances to purchase safety equipment or make repairs
        Lack of
            Safety education
            Safety precautions
        Language barrier
    External (Environmental)
        Bathing
            In very hot water
            Without hand grips
            Without anti-slip equipment
        Children
            Carried on adult bicycles
            Playing near vehicle pathways
            Playing with candles, cigarettes, matches, sharp-edged toys
            Playing without safety gates near stairs, unsupervised

Text continued on following page

High-Risk Diagnosis: *High Risk for Trauma*
(Continued)

Riding bicycles without headgear
Riding in front seat of car or without seat restraints
Contact with
    Acids or alkalis
    Dangerous machinery
    Intense cold
    Rapidly moving machinery, industrial belts, or
        pulleys
Driving
    After partaking of alcohol, drugs
    At excessive speeds
    Cycles without headgear
    Mechanically unsafe vehicle
    Without necessary visual aids
    Without seat restraints
Electrical hazards
    Faulty electrical plugs, frayed wires, or defective
        appliances
    Overloaded electrical outlets, fuse boxes
    Unanchored electrical wires
Fire hazards
    Experimenting with chemicals, gasoline
    Gas leaks, delayed lighting of burner or oven
    Grease waste collected on stoves
    Highly flammable toys, clothing
    Incorrectly stored combustibles or corrosives
    Playing with fireworks, gunpowder
    Pot handles facing front of stove
    Smoking in bed or near oxygen
    Unscreened fires or heaters
    Use of thin, worn potholders or mitts
    Wearing plastic flammable clothing
Safety hazards
    Entering unlighted rooms
    Guns or ammunition stored unlocked
    High beds
    High-crime neighborhood and vulnerable client
    Knives stored uncovered
    Large icicles hanging from roof
    Litter or liquids on floor, stairway
    Obstructed passageways
    Slippery floors
    Snow or ice on stairs, walkways

Unanchored rugs
Unsafe road or crossing
Unsafe window protection
Unsturdy or absent stair rails
Unsteady ladders, chairs
Use of cracked dishware, glasses
Miscellaneous
Inappropriate call-for-aid mechanism for client on
bedrest
Sliding on coarse bed linen
Struggling within bed restraints
Overexposure to sun, sunlamps, radiotherapy

High-Risk Diagnosis: *High Risk for Aspiration*

Definition: The state in which an individual is at risk for entry of gastrointestinal secretions, oropharyngeal secretions, solids, or fluids into tracheobronchial passages

Risk Factors

Reduced level of consciousness
Depressed cough and gag reflexes
Presence of tracheostomy or endotracheal tube
Incomplete lower esophageal sphincter
Gastrointestinal tubes
Tube feedings
Medication administration
Situations hindering elevation of upper body
Increased intragastric pressure
Increased gastric residual
Decreased gastrointestinal motility
Delayed gastric emptying
Impaired swallowing
Facial, oral, or neck surgery or trauma
Wired jaw

High-Risk Diagnosis: *High Risk for Disuse Syndrome*

Definition: The state in which an individual is at risk for deterioration of body systems as the result of prescribed or unavoidable musculoskeletal inactivity

Risk Factors

     Paralysis
     Mechanical immobilization
     Prescribed immobilization
     Severe pain
     Altered level of consciousness

Diagnosis: *Altered Protection*

Definition: The state in which an individual experiences a decrease in the ability to guard the self from internal or external threats such as illness or injury

Defining Characteristics

Major

Deficient immunity

Impaired healing

Altered clotting

Maladaptive stress response

Neurosensory alterations

Minor

Chilling

Perspiring

Dyspnea

Cough

Itching

Restlessness

Insomnia

Fatigue

Anorexia

Weakness

Immobility

Disorientation

Pressure sores

Related Factors

Effects of extremes of age

Inadequate nutrition

Alcohol abuse

Abnormal blood profiles (leukopenia, thrombocytopenia, anemia, coagulation)

Drug therapies (antineoplastic, corticosteroid, immune, anti-coagulant, thrombolytic)

Treatments (surgery, radiation)

Diseases (cancer, immune disorders)

Diagnosis: *Impaired Tissue Integrity*

Definition: The state in which an individual experiences damage to mucous membrane or corneal, integumentary, or subcutaneous tissue

Defining Characteristics
> Damaged or destroyed tissue
>> Cornea
>> Mucous membrane
>> Integumentary
>> Subcutaneous

Related Factors
> Altered circulation
> Effects of therapeutic radiation
> Fluid deficit/excess
> Impaired mobility
> Irritants
>> Chemical
>>> Body excretions
>>> Body secretions
>>> Medications
>> Mechanical
>>> Friction
>>> Pressure
>>> Shear
>> Thermal
>>> Temperature extremes
> Nutritional deficit/excess
> Knowledge deficit

Diagnosis: *Altered Oral Mucous Membrane*

Definition: The state in which an individual experiences disruption in the tissue layers of the oral cavity

Defining Characteristics
> Atrophy of gums
> Coated tongue
> Dry mouth (xerostomia)
> Edema of mucosa
> Halitosis
> Hemorrhagic gingivitis
> Hyperemia
> Lack of or decreased salivation
> Oral
>> Carious teeth
>> Desquamation
>> Lesions
>> Pain or discomfort
>> Plaque
>> Redness
>> Ulcers
>> Vesicles
> Stomatitis

Related Factors
> Dehydration
> Effects of
>> Chemotherapy
>> Medication
>> Radiation to head/neck
>> Surgery
> Immunosuppression
> Inadequate oral hygiene
> Infection
> Lack of or decreased salivation
> Mouth breathing
> Malnutrition/vitamin deficiency
> NPO for more than 24 hours
> Trauma
>> Chemical associated with
>>> Acidic foods
>>> Alcohol
>>> Drugs

Noxious agents
Tobacco
Mechanical associated with
Braces
Broken teeth
Endotracheal tube
Ill-fitting dentures
Nasogastric tube placement
Vomiting

Diagnosis: *Impaired Skin Integrity*

Definition: The state in which an individual experiences an alteration or disruption of the skin

Defining Characteristics
>Disruption of
>>Skin surface
>Invasion of body structures

Related Factors
>External
>>Chemical substance
>>Humidity
>>Hyperthermia
>>Hypothermia
>>Mechanical factors
>>>Shearing forces
>>>Pressure
>>>Restraints
>>Physical immobilization
>>Radiation
>Internal (somatic)
>>Altered
>>>Circulation
>>>Metabolic state
>>>Nutritional state
>>>>Emaciation
>>>>Obesity
>>>Pigmentation
>>>Sensation
>>>Turgor (change in elasticity)
>>Developmental factors
>>Effects of medication
>>Immunological deficit
>>Skeletal prominence

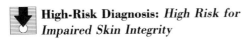 **High-Risk Diagnosis:** *High Risk for Impaired Skin Integrity*

Definition: The state in which an individual is at risk of experiencing an alteration or disruption of the skin

Risk Factors
    External
        Chemical substance
        Excretions or secretions
        Humidity
        Hyperthermia
        Hypothermia
        Mechanical factors
            Shearing forces
            Pressure
            Restraints
        Physical immobilization
        Radiation
    Internal (somatic)
        Altered
            Circulation
            Metabolic state
            Nutritional state
                Emaciation
                Obesity
            Pigmentation
            Sensation
            Turgor (change in elasticity)
        Developmental factors
        Effects of medication
        Immunological deficit
        Psychogenic
        Skeletal prominence

Communicating
A human response pattern involving sending messages

 Diagnosis: *Impaired Verbal Communication*

The state in which an individual experiences a decreased or absent ability to use or understand language in human interaction

Defining Characteristics
> Difficulty with phonation
> Disorientation
> Dyspnea
> Flight of ideas
> Impaired articulation
> Inability to
>> Find words
>> Identify objects
>> Modulate speech
>> Name words
>
> Lack of desire to speak, speak dominant language, speak in sentences
> Incessant verbalization
> Loose association of ideas
> Stuttering/slurring

Related Factors
> Altered thought processes
> Auditory impairment
> Decreased circulation to the brain
> Effects of
>> Surgery
>> Trauma
>
> Inflammation
> Mental retardation
> Oral deformities
> Physical barrier
>> Intubation
>> Tracheostomy
>
> Respiratory embarrassment
> Speech pattern dysfunction
> Inability to read or write
> Ineffective listening skills
> Language barrier
> Psychological barriers
>> Anxiety
>> Fear

Relating

A human response pattern involving established bonds

 Diagnosis: *Impaired Social Interaction*

Definition: The state in which an individual participates in an insufficient or excessive quantity or ineffective quality of social exchange

Defining Characteristics
Major

Verbalized or observed discomfort

In social situations

In receiving or communicating a satisfying sense of belonging, caring, interest, or shared history

Observed use of unsuccessful socialization behaviors

Dysfunctional interaction with peers, family, and/or others

Minor

Family report of change of style or pattern of interaction

Related Factors
Knowledge/skills deficit about ways to enhance mutuality

Communication barriers

Self-concept disturbances

Absence of available significant others or peers

Limited physical mobility

Therapeutic isolation

Sociocultural dissonance

Environmental barriers

Diagnosis: *Social Isolation*

Definition: The state in which an individual experiences aloneness that is perceived as imposed by others and as negative or threatening

Defining Characteristics

    Objective

        Absence of supportive significant other(s) (family, friends, group)

        Sad, dull affect

        Inappropriate or immature interests/activities for developmental age/stage

        Uncommunicative, withdrawn, no eye contact

        Preoccupation with own thoughts; repetitive, meaningless actions

        Projects hostility in voice, behavior

        Seeks to be alone or exists in a subculture

        Evidence of physical/mental handicap or altered state of wellness

        Shows behavior unaccepted by dominant cultural group

    Subjective

        Expresses feelings of

            Aloneness imposed by others

            Rejection

        Experiences feelings of difference from others

        Inadequacy in or absence of significant purpose in life

        Inability to meet expectations of others

        Insecurity in public

        Expresses

            Values acceptable to the subculture but unacceptable to the dominant cultural group

            Interests inappropriate to the developmental age/state

Related Factors

    Factors contributing to the absence of satisfying personal relationships such as

        Delay in accomplishing developmental tasks

        Immature interests

        Alterations in

            Mental status

            Physical appearance

            State of wellness

Unacceptable
    Social behavior
    Values
Inability to engage in satisfying personal relationships
Inadequate personal resources
Inadequate support systems
    Living alone
    Recent retirement
    Recent/frequent change of residence
    Loss of a significant other
Stress

Diagnosis: *Altered Role Performance*

Definition: The state in which an individual experiences a change, conflict, or denial of role responsibilities or inability to perform role responsibilities

Defining Characteristics
> Changes in
>> Self-perception of role
>> Others' perception of role
>> Physical capacity to resume role
>> Usual patterns of responsibility
> Conflicts in roles
> Disparity between self and others in defining roles
> Denial of role
> Lack of knowledge of role
> Observed difficulty performing role function
> States inability to perform role expectations

Related Factors
> Change in
>> Employment
>> Family structure
>> Financial status
>> Health status
> Combination of role loss and acquisition
> Cultural transition
> Developmental crisis
> Ineffective coping mechanisms
> Loss of support group
> Role acquisition
> Role loss

Diagnosis: *Altered Parenting*

Definition: The state in which a nuturing figure(s) experiences inability to create an environment which promotes optimal growth and development of another human being

Defining Characteristics
> Abandonment
> Runaway
> Verbalizes
>> Inability to control child
>> Disappointment in gender or physical characteristics of an infant/child (constant)
>> Resentment toward infant/child
>> Role inadequacy
>> Frustration
>> Disgust at body functions of infant/child
>> Desire to have child call him/her by first name versus traditional cultural tendencies
> Lack of parental attachment behaviors
> Inappropriate visual, tactile, auditory stimulation
> Negative
>> Identification of infant's/child's characteristics
>> Attachment of meanings to infant's/child's characteristics
> Inattention to infant's/child's needs
> Inappropriate caretaking behaviors
>> Toilet training
>> Sleep and rest
>> Feeding
> Noncompliance with health appointments for infant/child
> Inappropriate or inconsistent discipline practices
> Frequent
>> Accidents
>> Illnesses
> Growth and development lag in child
> History of child abuse or abandonment by primary caretaker
> Child receives care from multiple caretakers without consideration of the needs of the infant/child
> Compulsively seeks role approval from others

Related Factors
> Ineffective role model
> Effects of
>> Physical and psychosocial abuse of nurturing figure

Text continued on following page

Diagnosis: *Altered Parenting (Continued)*

        Unmet social/emotional maturational needs of parenting
           figures
        Interruption in bonding process, i.e., maternal, paternal,
           other
        Unrealistic expectations for self, infant, partner
        Intensive or special care requirements
        Multiple pregnancies
        Physical or mental handicaps
        Acute/chronic mental or physical illnesses
        Limited cognitive functioning
    Lack of
        Available role model
        Support between/from significant other(s)
        Knowledge
        Role identity
        Or inappropriate response of child to relationship
    Perceived threat to own survival, physical and emotional
    Presence of stress (financial, legal, recent crisis, cultural
        move)

High-Risk Diagnosis: *High Risk for Altered Parenting*

Definition: The state in which a nurturing figure(s) is at risk to experience an inability to create an environment that promotes the optimal growth and development of another human being

Risk Factors

Ineffective role model
Effects of
Physical and psychosocial abuse of nurturing figure
Unmet social/emotional maturational needs of parenting figures
Interruption in bonding process, i.e., maternal, paternal, other
Unrealistic expectations for self, infant, partner
Intensive or special care requirements
Multiple pregnancies
Physical or mental handicaps
Acute/chronic mental or physical illnesses
Limited cognitive functioning
Lack of
Available role model
Support between/from significant other(s)
Knowledge
Role identity
Or inappropriate response of child to relationship
Perceived threat to own survival, physical and emotional
Presence of stress (financial, legal, recent crisis, cultural move)

Diagnosis: *Sexual Dysfunction*

Definition: The state in which an individual experiences a change in sexual function that is viewed as unsatisfying, unrewarding, or inadequate

Defining Characteristics
>Verbalization of problem
>Alterations in
>>Achieving perceived sex role
>>Achieving sexual satisfaction
>>Relationship with significant other
>Actual or perceived limitation imposed by disease and/or therapy
>Conflicts involving values
>Inability to achieve desired satisfaction
>Seeking confirmation of desirability
>Change of interest in self and others

Related Factors
>Biopsychosocial alteration of sexuality
>>Ineffective or absent role models
>>Physical abuse
>>Psychosocial abuse, e.g., harmful relationships
>>Vulnerability
>>Values conflict
>>Lack of
>>>Privacy
>>>Significant other
>>>Knowledge
>>Effects of altered body structure/function
>>>Pregnancy
>>>Recent childbirth
>>>Drugs
>>>Surgery
>>>Anomalies
>>>Disease process
>>>Trauma
>>>Radiation
>>Misinformation

Diagnosis: *Altered Family Processes*

Definition: The state in which a family that normally functions effectively experiences a dysfunction

Defining Characteristics

Family system unable or unwilling to

Meet physical, spiritual, security, emotional needs of all its members

Communicate openly and effectively

Express or accept a wide range of feelings from other family members

Relate to each other for mutual growth and maturation

Demonstrate flexibility in function and roles

Demonstrate respect for individuality and autonomy of its members

Accomplish current or past developmental tasks

Make effective decisions

Become involved in community activities

Seek or accept help appropriately

Adapt to change or deal with traumatic experience constructively

Presence of inappropriate or poorly communicated

Direction and level of energy

Family rules, rituals, or symbols

Related Factors

Situational or developmental transitions and/or crises

Reduced income

Unemployment

Relocation

Large number of family members

Multigenerational family

Single-parent family

Loss or gain of significant other

Conflict or change in family role

Absent or ineffective family role models

Effects of chronic illness

Diagnosis: *Caregiver Role Strain*

Definition: A caregiver's felt difficulty in performing the family caregiver role

Defining Characteristics
Caregivers report that they
>Do not have enough resources to provide the care needed
>Find it hard to do specific caregiving activities
>Worry about such issues as the care receiver's health and emotional state, having to put the care receiver in an institution, and who will care for the individual if something should happen to the caregiver

Feel that caregiving interferes with other important roles in their lives

Feel loss because the care receiver is like a different person, compared with before caregiving began, or in the case of a child, feel that he/she was never the child the caregiver expected

Feel family conflict related to issues of providing care

Feel stress or nervousness in their relationship with the care receiver

Feel depressed

Related Factors
Pathophysiological/Physiological
>Illness severity of the care receiver
>Addiction or codependency
>Premature birth/congenital defect
>Discharge of family member with significant home care needs
>Caregiver health impairment
>Caregiver is female

Developmental
>Caregiver is not developmentally ready for caregiver role, e.g., young adult needed to provide care for a middle-aged parent
>Developmental delay or retardation of the care receiver or caregiver

Psychosocial
>Psychological or cognitive problems in the care receiver
>Marginal family adaptation or dysfunction prior to caregiving situation
>Marginal caregiver's coping patterns

Past history of poor relationship between caregiver and care receiver

Caregiver is spouse

Care receiver exhibits deviant, bizarre behavior

Situational

Presence of abuse or violence

Presence of situational stressors that normally affect families, such as significant loss; disaster or crisis; poverty or economic vulnerability; major life events, e.g., birth, hospitalization, leaving home, returning home, marriage, divorce, employment, retirement, death

Duration of caregiving required

Inadequate physical environment for providing care, e.g., housing, transportation, community services, equipment

Family/caregiver isolation

Lack of respite and recreation for caregiver

Inexperience with caregiving

Caregiver's competing role commitments

Complexity/amount of caregiving tasks

High-Risk Diagnosis: *High Risk for Caregiver Role Strain*

Definition: A caregiver is vulnerable for felt difficulty in performing the family caregiver role

Risk Factors

Pathophysiological

Illness severity of the care receiver

Addiction or codependency

Premature birth/congenital defect

Discharge of family member with significant home care needs

Caregiver health impairment

Unpredictable illness course or instability in the care receiver's health

Caregiver is female

Psychological or cognitive problems in the care receiver

Developmental

Caregiver is not developmentally ready for caregiver role, e.g., young adult needed to provide care for a middle-aged parent

Developmental delay or retardation of the care receiver or caregiver

Psychosocial

Marginal family adaptation or dysfunction prior to caregiving situation

Marginal caregiver's coping patterns

Past history of poor relationship between caregiver and care receiver

Caregiver is spouse

Care receiver exhibits deviant, bizarre behavior

Situational

Presence of abuse or violence

Presence of situational stressors that normally affect families, such as significant loss; disaster or crisis; poverty or economic vulnerability; major life events, e.g., birth, hospitalization, leaving home, returning home, marriage, divorce, employment, retirement, death

Duration of caregiving required

Inadequate physical environment for providing care, e.g., housing, transportation, community services, equipment

Family/caregiver isolation
Lack of respite and recreation for caregiver
Inexperience with caregiving
Caregiver's competing role commitments
Complexity/amount of caregiving tasks

Diagnosis: *Parental Role Conflict*

Definition: The state in which a parent experiences role confusion and conflict in response to a crisis

Defining Characteristics
Major

Parent(s) expresses

Concerns/feelings of inadequacy to provide for child's physical and emotional needs during hospitalization or in the home

Concerns about changes in parental role, family functioning, family communication, family health

Demonstrated disruption in caretaking routines

Minor

Expresses concern about perceived loss of control over decisions relating to child

Reluctant to participate in usual caretaking activities, even with encouragement and support

Verbalizes/demonstrates feelings of guilt, anger, fear, anxiety, and/or frustration about effect of child's illness on family process

Related Factors
Separation from child because of chronic illness

Intimidation with invasive or restrictive modalities (isolation, intubation), specialized care centers, policies

Home care of a child with special needs (apnea monitoring, postural drainage, hyperalimentation)

Interruptions of family life because of home care regimen (treatments, caregivers, lack of respite)

Change in marital status

Diagnosis: *Altered Sexuality Patterns*

Definition: The state in which individuals express concern regarding their sexuality

Defining Characteristics
Major: Reported difficulties, limitations, or changes in sexual behaviors or activities

Related Factors
Effects of illness or medical treatment
  Drugs
  Radiation
  Anomalies
Extreme fatigue
Obesity
Pain
Performance anxiety
Knowledge/skill deficit about alternative responses to health-related transitions
  Pregnancy
  Surgery
  Recent childbirth
  Trauma
  Menopause
Impaired relationship with a significant other
Lack of significant other
Fear of pregnancy or of acquiring a sexually transmitted disease
Conflicts with sexual orientation or variant preferences
Ineffective or absent role models
Loss of job or ability to work
Separation from or loss of significant other

Valuing

A human response pattern involving the assigning of relative worth

 Diagnosis: *Spiritual Distress*

Definition: The state in which an individual experiences a disruption in the life principle that pervades a person's entire being and that integrates and transcends one's biological and psychosocial nature

Defining Characteristics

Self-destructive behavior or threats
Alteration in behavior or mood evidenced by anger, crying, preoccupation, anxiety, hostility
Sleep pattern disturbances
Feeling separated or alienated from deity
Feelings of helplessness or hopelessness
Depression
Expresses concerns about meaning of life and death and/or belief systems
Verbalizes inner conflict about beliefs
Questions moral and ethical implications of therapeutic regimen
Inability to participate in usual religious practices
Regards illness as punishment
Requests spiritual assistance for a disturbance in belief system
Displacement of anger toward clergy
Does not experience that God is forgiving
Engages in self-blame

Related Factors

Loss of significant others
Challenged belief and value system, e.g., result of moral or ethical implications associated with disease process, therapy, or intense suffering
Beliefs opposed by family, peers, or health care providers
Disruption in usual religious activity
Effects of personal and family disasters or major life changes

Choosing
A human response pattern involving the selection of alternatives

 Diagnosis: *Ineffective Individual Coping*

Definition: The state in which an individual demonstrates impaired adaptive behaviors and problem-solving abilities in meeting life's demands and roles

Defining Characteristics
> Insomnia
> Physical inactivity
> Stress-related disorders
>> Ulcers
>> Hypertension
>> Irritable bowel
> Substance abuse
> Inappropriate use of defense mechanisms
>> Withdrawal
>> Depression
>> Overeating
>> Blaming
>> Scapegoating
>> Manipulative behavior
>> Self-pity
> Change in usual communication patterns
> Inability to meet or take responsibility for basic needs
> Chronic anxiety
> Exaggerated fear of pain, death
> General irritability
> Fear of pain, death
> Inability to problem solve
> High rate of accidents or illnesses
> Frequent headaches/neckaches
> Emotional tension
> Verbalizes inability to cope or inability to ask for help
> Use of magical thinking
> Inability to perform expected roles
> Indecisiveness
> Violence toward others
> Self-destructive behavior
> Unfamiliar environment

Text continued on following page

Diagnosis: *Ineffective Individual Coping (Continued)*

Related Factors
Effects of acute or chronic illness
Loss of control over body part or body function
Lack of support systems
Separation from or loss of significant other
Low self-esteem
Major changes in lifestyle
Unrealistic perceptions
Situational or maturational crises
Inadequate leisure activities
Knowledge deficit regarding
    Therapeutic regimen
    Disease process
    Prognosis
Sensory overload

Diagnosis: *Impaired Adjustment*

Definition: The state in which the individual is unable to modify lifestyle/behavior in a manner consistent with a change in health status

Defining Characteristics
Verbalizes nonacceptance of health status change
Extended period of shock, disbelief, or anger regarding health status change
Lack of future-oriented thinking
Nonexistent or unsuccessful ability to be involved in problem solving or goal setting
Lack of movement toward independence

Related Factors
Effects of disability requiring change in lifestyle
Sensory overload
Impaired cognition
Incomplete grieving
Assault to self-esteem
Altered locus of control
Inadequate support systems

Diagnosis: *Defensive Coping*

Definition: The state in which an individual repeatedly projects falsely positive self-evaluation based on a self-protective pattern that defends against underlying perceived threats to positive self-regard

Defining Characteristics
Major

Denial of obvious problems/weaknesses
Projection of blame/responsibility
Rationalization of failures
Hypersensitivity to slight criticism
Grandiosity

Minor

Superior attitude toward others
Difficulty establishing/maintaining relationships
Hostile laughter or ridicule of others
Difficulty in reality-testing perceptions
Lack of follow-through or participation in treatment or therapy

Diagnosis: *Ineffective Denial*

Definition: The state in which an individual consciously or unconsciously attempts to disavow the knowledge or meaning of an event to reduce anxiety/fear to the detriment of health

Defining Characteristics
> Major
>> Delays in seeking or refuses health care attention to the detriment of health
>> Does not perceive personal relevance of symptoms or danger
>
> Minor
>> Uses home remedies (self-treatment) to relieve symptoms
>> Does not admit fear of death or invalidism
>> Minimizes symptoms
>> Displaces source of symptoms to other organs
>> Unable to admit impact of disease on life pattern
>> Makes dismissive gestures or comments when speaking of distressing events
>> Displaces fear of impact of the condition
>> Displays inappropriate affect

Diagnosis: *Ineffective Family Coping: Disabling*

Definition: The state in which the behavior of a significant person (family member or other primary person) disables their capacities to address effectively tasks essential to either person's adaptation to a health challenge

Defining Characteristics

Assumption of dependency role
Excessive vigilance over family member
Adopting symptoms/signs of ill family member
Denial of existence or severity of illness of family member
Exploitation or neglect of family members
Child, spousal, or elder abuse
Despair
Unresolved anger or depression
Rejection or desertion
Intolerance
Impaired decision making
Substance abuse

Related Factors

Effects of major life events
Major changes in social/cultural environment
Effects of recent or impending death of family member
Marital discord
Chronically unexpressed feelings of guilt, despair, anxiety, or hostility
Highly ambivalent family relationships
Dissonant discrepancy of coping styles
Unmet psychosocial needs of child or parent
Lack of economic resources or support systems

Diagnosis: *Ineffective Family Coping: Compromised*

Definition: The state in which a usually supportive primary person (family member or close friend) is providing insufficient, ineffective, or compromised support, comfort, assistance, or encouragement that may be needed by the client to manage or master adaptive tasks related to a health challenge

Defining Characteristics

Ineffective responses to illness, disability, or situational crises

Withdrawal

Overprotection

Preoccupation with personal reactions, i.e., blaming or scapegoating

Manipulative behaviors

Inability to demonstrate supportive behaviors

Expressed concern about significant other's response to health problem

Impaired intimacy or closeness

Attempted assistive behaviors with less than satisfactory results

Related Factors

Isolation of family members from one another

Lack of support for family members

Temporary family disorganization and role changes

Effects of acute or chronic illness

Incompatible or differing values, beliefs, or goals

Unrealistic expectations

Knowledge deficit

Temporary preoccupation resulting in inability to perceive or act effectively in regard to health needs

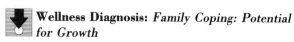 **Wellness Diagnosis:** *Family Coping: Potential for Growth*

Definition: Effective managing of adaptive tasks by family member involved with the client's health challenge, who now is exhibiting desire and readiness for enhanced health and growth in regard to self and in relation to the client

Defining Characteristics

Family members attempt to describe growth impact of crises on their own values, priorities, goals, or relationships

Individual expresses interest in making contact on a one-to-one basis or on a mutual and group basis with another person who has experienced a similar situation

Family member is moving in direction of health-promoting and enriching lifestyle that supports and monitors maturational processes, audits and negotiates treatment programs, and generally chooses experiences that optimize wellness

Related Factors

The family's basic needs are sufficiently gratified and adaptive tasks effectively addressed to enable goals of self-actualization to surface

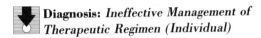 **Diagnosis:** *Ineffective Management of Therapeutic Regimen (Individual)*

Definition: A pattern of regulating and integrating into daily living a program for treatment of illness and the sequelae of illness that is unsatisfactory for meeting specific health goals

Defining Characteristics

Major

Choices of daily living ineffective for meeting the goals of a treatment or prevention program

Minor

Acceleration (expected or unexpected) of illness symptoms

Verbalized desire to manage the treatment of illness and prevention of sequelae

Verbalized difficulty with regulation/integration of one or more prescribed regimens for treatment of illness and its effects or prevention of complications

Verbalized that did not take action to include treatment regimens in daily routines

Verbalized that did not take action to reduce risk factors for progression of illness and sequelae

Related Factors

Complexity of health care system

Complexity of therapeutic regimen

Decisional conflicts

Economic difficulties

Excessive demands made on individual or family

Family conflict

Family patterns of health care

Inadequate number and types of cues to action

Knowledge deficits

Mistrust of regimen and/or health care personnel

Perceived seriousness

Perceived susceptibility

Perceived barriers

Perceived benefits

Powerlessness

Social support deficits

Diagnosis: *Noncompliance (Specify)*

Definition: The state in which an individual makes an informed decision not to adhere to a therapeutic recommendation

Defining Characteristics

Observed or reported

Evidence of development of complications
Evidence of exacerbation of symptoms
Failure to progress
Clinical data (blood/urine levels)
Failure to resolve health problems
Nonadherence to therapeutic regimen
Nonadherence after education
Failure to keep appointments
Inability to set or attain mutual goals
Failure to seek care when disease status warrants

Related Factors

Side effects of medications
Impaired ability to perform tasks
Concurrent illness of family member
Increasing amount of disease-related symptoms despite adherence to advised regimen
Denial
Depression
Forgetfulness
Feeling of lack of control
Knowledge deficit
Lack of perceived benefits of treatment
Cultural or spiritual values
Complexity of therapeutic regimen
Client and provider relationships
Previous unsuccessful experience with advised regimen
Lack of support system
Lack of economic resources (money, transportation)

Diagnosis: *Decisional Conflict (Specify)*

Definition: The state in which an individual experiences uncertainty about the course of action to be taken when choice among competing actions involves risk, loss, or challenge to personal life values

Defining Characteristics
Major

Verbalized uncertainty about choices

Verbalized undesired consequences of alternative actions being considered

Vacillation among alternative choices

Delayed decision making

Minor

Verbalized feelings of distress while attempting a decision

Self-focusing

Physical signs of distress or tension (increased heart rate, increased muscle tension, restlessness)

Questioning personal values and beliefs while attempting a decision

Related Factors
Unclear personal values/beliefs

Perceived threat to value system

Lack of experience or interference with decision making

Lack of relevant information

Multiple or divergent sources of information

Support system deficit

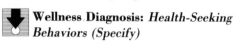

Wellness Diagnosis: *Health-Seeking Behaviors (Specify)*

Definition: The state in which an individual in stable health is actively seeking ways to alter personal health habits and/or the environment in order to move toward a higher level of health (stable health status is defined as follows: age-appropriate illness prevention measures are achieved, client reports good or excellent health, and signs and symptoms of disease, if present, are controlled)

Defining Characteristics
> Major
>> Expressed or observed desire to seek a higher level of wellness
> Minor
>> Expressed or observed desire for increased control of health practice
>> Expressed concern about current environmental conditions on health status
>> Stated or observed unfamiliarity with wellness community resources
>> Demonstrated or observed lack of knowledge in health promotion behaviors

Moving
A human response pattern involving activity

 Diagnosis: *Impaired Physical Mobility*

Definition: The state in which an individual experiences limitation of ability needed for independent physical movement

Defining Characteristics
Reluctance to attempt movement
Imposed restrictions on movement
Limited range of motion
Decreased muscle strength, control, and/or mass
Inability to move purposefully within the physical environment, including bed mobility, transfer, and ambulation
Impaired coordination
Falling or stumbling

Related Factors
Neuromuscular impairment
Sensory-perceptual impairment
Fatigue, decreased strength and endurance
Intolerance to activity
Effects of
> Neuromuscular impairment
> Sensory-perceptual impairment
> Trauma or surgery

Inflammation
Pain
Obesity
Side effects of sedatives, narcotics, or tranquilizers
Depression
Severe anxiety
Fear of movement
Architectural barriers
Lack of assistive devices

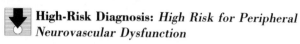

High-Risk Diagnosis: *High Risk for Peripheral Neurovascular Dysfunction*

Definition: A state in which an individual is at risk of experiencing a disruption in circulation, sensation, or motion of an extremity

Risk Factors
    Fractures
    Mechanical compression, e.g., tourniquet, cast, brace, dressing, or restraint
    Orthopedic surgery
    Trauma
    Immobilization
    Burns
    Vascular obstruction

Diagnosis: *Activity Intolerance*

Definition: The state in which an individual has insufficient physiological or psychological energy to endure or complete required or desired daily activities

Defining Characteristics
> Increased or decreased heart rate, blood pressure, respirations
> Electrocardiographic changes reflecting dysrhythmias or ischemia
> Exertional discomfort or dyspnea
> Redness, cyanosis, or pallor of skin during activity
> Dizziness during activity
> Impaired ability to change position or stand or walk without support
> Weakness
> Requiring frequent rest periods
> Worried or uneasy facial expression
> Verbal report of fatigue or weakness
> Confusion

Related Factors
> Electrolyte imbalance
> Hypovolemia
> Malnourishment
> Interrupted sleep
> Impaired sensory or motor function
> Deconditioned status
> Imbalance between oxygen supply and demand
> Effects of
>> Aging
>> Impaired sensory or motor function
>> Medications (sedatives, tranquilizers, narcotics)
> Generalized weakness
> Pain
> Fatigue
> Bedrest
> Immobility
> Depression
> Lack of motivation
> Sedentary lifestyle

Diagnosis: *Fatigue*

Definition: The state in which an individual experiences an overwhelming sense of exhaustion and decreased capacity for physical and mental work

Defining Characteristics
Major
> Verbalization of an unremitting and overwhelming lack of energy
> Inability to maintain usual routines

Minor
> Perceived need for additional energy to accomplish routine tasks
> Increase in physical complaints
> Impaired ability to concentrate
> Decreased performance
> Lethargy or listlessness
> Disinterest in surroundings/introspection
> Decreased libido
> Accident-prone
> Emotionally labile or irritable

Related Factors
Decreased/increased metabolic energy production
Increased energy requirements to perform activities of daily living
Overwhelming psychological or emotional demands
Excessive social and/or role demands
States of discomfort
Altered body chemistry
> Medications
> Drug withdrawal
> Chemotherapy

High-Risk Diagnosis: *High Risk for Activity Intolerance*

Definition: The state in which an individual is at risk of experiencing insufficient physiological or psychological energy to endure or complete required or desired daily activities

Risk Factors

History of previous intolerance
Deconditioned status
Presence of circulatory/respiratory problems
Inexperience with the activity

Diagnosis: *Sleep Pattern Disturbance*

Definition: The state in which disruption of sleep time causes discomfort or interferes with desired lifestyle

Defining Characteristics
>Verbal complaints of
>>Difficulty falling asleep
>>Awakening earlier or later than desired
>>Interrupted sleep
>>Not feeling well-rested
>Changes in behavior or performance; increasing
>>Irritability
>>Restlessness
>>Disorientation
>>Lethargy
>>Listlessness
>Physical signs
>>Mild fleeting nystagmus
>>Slight hand tremor
>>Ptosis of eyelid
>>Expressionless face
>>Headache
>>Dark circles under eyes, reddened eyes
>>Frequent yawning
>>Changes in posture
>Thick speech with mispronunciation and incorrect words
>Napping during day
>Mood alterations
>Difficulty in concentration

Related Factors
>Effects of
>>Pregnancy
>>Medications
>>Sensory alterations
>>>Internal (illness, psychological stress)
>>>External (environmental changes, social cues)
>Pain
>Inactivity
>Diarrhea
>Urinary frequency
>Incontinence
>Nausea

Lifestyle disruptions
Demands of caring for others
Stress
Fear or anxiety
Depression
Nightmares
Sensory overload
Unfamiliar environment
Circadian rhythm disturbances (shift work)

Diagnosis: *Diversional Activity Deficit*

Definition: The state in which an individual experiences a decreased stimulation from or interest or engagement in recreational or leisure activities

Defining Characteristics

    Weight loss or gain
    Yawning
    Crying
    Restlessness
    Preoccupation with self
    Napping during day
    Apathy or hostility
    Complaints of boredom
    Verbalizations of desire for activity
    Depression
    Inability to participate in usual hobbies because of physical limitations or hospitalization

Related Factors

    Effects of chronic illness
    Frequent, lengthy treatments
    Unwillingness to learn new skills or acquire new interests
    Social isolation
    Confined to bedrest
    Preoccupation with job
    Decreased economic resources

Diagnosis: *Impaired Home Maintenance Management*

Definition: The state in which an individual experiences the inability to maintain independently a safe, growth-producing immediate environment

Defining Characteristics
    Subjective
        Household members
            Express difficulty in maintaining home in a comfortable fashion
            Request assistance with home maintenance
            Describe outstanding debt or financial crisis
    Objective
        Disorderly surroundings
        Unwashed or unavailable
            Cooking equipment
            Clothes
            Linen
        Offensive odors
        Presence of rodents or vermin
        Inappropriate household temperature
        Accumulation of
            Dirt
            Food wastes
            Hygienic wastes
        Overtaxed family members (exhausted, anxious)
        Lack of necessary equipment or aids
        Repeated
            Hygienic disorders
            Infestations
            Infections

Related Factors
    Individual/family member disease or injury
    Impaired mental status
    Substance abuse
    Effects of chronic debilitating disease
    Depression
    Lack of
        Knowledge
        Motivation
        Role modeling
    Decreased financial resources

Text continued on following page

Diagnosis: *Impaired Home Maintenance Management (Continued)*

Insufficient
    Family organization or planning
    Finances
Inadequate support systems
Unfamiliarity with neighborhood resources

Diagnosis: *Altered Health Maintenance*

Definition: The state in which an individual experiences inability to identify, manage, and/or seek out help to maintain health status

Defining Characteristics

Demonstrated lack of

Knowledge regarding basic health practices

Adaptive behaviors to internal or external environmental changes

Reported or observed

Inability to take responsibility for meeting basic health practices in any or all functional pattern areas

Lack of equipment, financial, and/or other resources

Impairment of personal support systems

History of

lack of health-seeking behavior

Expressed interest in improving health behaviors

Failure to schedule routine examinations or immunizations

Failure to adjust lifestyle to demands of chronic or acute illness

Related Factors

Learning disability

Knowledge deficit

Stress

Substance abuse

Unachieved developmental tasks

Dysfunctional grieving

Ineffective individual or family coping

Lack of or significant alteration in

Communication skills (written, verbal, and/or gestural)

Ability to make deliberate and thoughtful judgments

Motivation

Support systems

Effects of perceptual/cognitive impairment (complete/ partial lack of gross and/or fine motor skills)

Ineffective individual/family coping

Dysfunctional grieving

Unachieved developmental tasks

Disabling spiritual distress

Lack of material resources

Feelings of helplessness

Fear of the unknown

Religious or cultural values

Loss of independence

Inaccessibility of adequate health care services

Diagnosis: *Feeding Self-Care Deficit*

Definition: The state in which an individual experiences impaired ability to perform or complete feeding activities for self

Defining Characteristics
> Inability to bring food from a receptacle to the mouth
> Inability to cut food
> Spilled food
> Untouched food
> Weight loss

Related Factors
> Effects of
>> Aging
>> Chronic illness
>> Cognitive/perceptual/neurovascular impairment
>> Loss of limbs
>> Medications
>> Trauma
>> Surgery
>> Visual impairment
> Lack of
>> Coordination
>> Motivation
>> Self-confidence
> Muscular weakness
> Fatigue
> Pain, discomfort
> Contractures
> Stiffness
> Presence of external devices—IV lines, casts, slings, traction, splints, restraints
> Immobility
> Psychotic states
> Depression
> Knowledge deficit
> Confusion
> Anxiety
> Grieving
> Dependency

Diagnosis: *Impaired Swallowing*

Definition: The state in which an individual has decreased ability to pass fluids and/or solids voluntarily from the mouth to the stomach

Defining Characteristics

Major

Observed evidence of difficulty in swallowing
Stasis of food in oral cavity
Regurgitation of fluids and/or solids through mouth or nose
Choking/coughing

Minor

Evidence of aspiration
Reported pain on swallowing
Dehydration
Weight loss

Related Factors

Effects of

Neuromuscular impairment
Decreased or absent gag reflex
Decreased strength or excursion of muscles of mastication

Perceptual impairment
Facial paralysis

Mechanical obstruction
Edema
Tracheostomy tube
Tumor

Excessive/inadequate salivation
Fatigue
Reddened, irritated oropharyngeal cavity
Limited awareness

Diagnosis: *Ineffective Breastfeeding*

Definition: The state in which a mother, infant, or child experiences dissatisfaction or difficulty with the breastfeeding process

Defining Characteristics
Major
> Unsatisfactory breastfeeding process

Minor
> Actual or perceived inadequate milk supply
> Infant inability to attach correctly onto maternal breast
> No observable signs of oxytocin release
> Observable signs of inadequate infant intake
> Nonsustained suckling at the breast
> Insufficient emptying of each breast per feeding
> Persistence of sore nipples beyond first week of breastfeeding
> Insufficient opportunity for suckling at the breast
> Infant exhibiting fussiness and crying within first hour after breastfeeding, unresponsive to other comfort measures
> Infant arching and crying at the breast, resisting latching on

Related Factors
> Infant anomaly
> Prematurity
> Maternal breast anomaly
> Previous breast surgery
> Previous history of breastfeeding failure
> Infant receiving supplemental feedings with artificial nipple
> Poor infant sucking reflex
> Nonsupportive partner/family
> Knowledge deficit
> Interruption to breastfeeding
> Maternal anxiety or ambivalence

Diagnosis: *Interrupted Breastfeeding*

Definition: A break in the continuity of the breastfeeding process as a result of inability or inadvisability of putting baby to breast for feeding

Defining Characteristics

Major

Infant does not receive nourishment at the breast for some or all of feedings

Minor

Maternal desire to maintain lactation and provide (or eventually provide) her breast milk for her infant's nutritional needs

Separation of mother and infant

Lack of knowledge regarding expression and storage of breast milk

Related Factors

Maternal or infant illness

Prematurity

Maternal employment

Contraindications to breastfeeding (e.g., drugs, true breast milk jaundice)

Need to wean infant abruptly

Wellness Diagnosis: *Effective Breastfeeding*

Definition: The state in which a mother-infant dyad/family exhibits adequate proficiency and satisfaction with the breastfeeding process

Defining Characteristics

Major

Mother able to position infant at breast to promote a successful latch-on response

Infant is content after feedings

Regular and sustained suckling/swallowing at the breast

Adequate infant weight gain

Minor

Signs and/or symptoms of oxytocin release (let down or milk ejection reflex)

Soft stools

Over six wet diapers per day of unconcentrated urine

Eagerness of infant to nurse

Maternal/family verbalization of satisfaction with the breastfeeding process

Related Factors

Basic breastfeeding knowledge

Normal breast structure

Normal infant oral structure

Infant gestational age greater than 34 weeks

Support sources

Maternal confidence

Diagnosis: *Ineffective Infant Feeding Pattern*

Definition: A state in which an infant demonstrates an impaired ability to suck or coordinate the suck-swallow response

Defining Characteristics
> Major
>> Inability to initiate or sustain an effective suck
>> Inability to coordinate sucking, swallowing, and breathing
>
> Minor
>> None

Related Factors
> Prematurity
> Neurological impairment/delay
> Oral hypersensitivity
> Prolonged NPO
> Anatomical abnormality
> Maternal confidence

Diagnosis: *Bathing/Hygiene Self-Care Deficit*

Definition: The state in which an individual experiences impaired ability to perform or complete bathing/hygiene activities for self

Defining Characteristics
> Dirt or stains on body
> Requests help in bathing
> Body odor
> Halitosis
> Inability to
>> Obtain or get to water source
>> Regulate water temperature or flow
>> Wash body or body parts

Related Factors
> Effects of
>> Aging
>> Chronic illness
>> Cognitive/perceptual impairment
>> Loss of limbs
>> Medications
>> Musculoskeletal/neuromuscular impairment
>> Surgery
>> Trauma
>> Visual impairment
> Lack of
>> Coordination
>> Motivation
>> Self-confidence
> Muscular weakness
> Fatigue
> Pain, discomfort
> Contractures
> Stiffness
> Presence of external devices—IV lines, casts, slings, traction, splints, restraints
> Immobility
> Psychotic states
> Depression
> Knowledge deficit
> Confusion
> Anxiety
> Grieving
> Dependency
> Intolerance to activity
> Decreased strength, endurance

Diagnosis: *Dressing/Grooming Self-Care Deficit*

Definition: The state in which an individual experiences impaired ability to perform or complete dressing and grooming activities for self

Defining Characteristics
Unshaven face
Uncombed hair
Unfastened clothes
Untied shoes
Overgrown fingernails and toenails
Wearing pajamas during day or daytime clothes to sleep in
Inability to
Maintain appearance at satisfactory level
Obtain, replace, or wash clothes
Put on or take off necessary items of clothing
Fasten clothing

Related Factors
Effects of
Aging
Chronic illness
Cognitive/perceptual impairment
Loss of limbs
Medications
Neuromuscular/musculoskeletal impairment
Surgery
Trauma
Visual impairment
Lack of
Coordination
Motivation
Self-confidence
Muscular weakness
Fatigue
Pain, discomfort
Contractures
Stiffness
Presence of external devices—IV lines, casts, slings, traction, splints, restraints
Immobility
Psychotic states
Depression
Knowledge deficit
Confusion

Text continued on following page

Diagnosis: *Dressing/Grooming Self-Care Deficit* *(Continued)*

Anxiety
Grieving
Dependency
Intolerance to activity
Decreased strength and endurance

Diagnosis: *Toileting Self-Care Deficit*

Definition: The state in which an individual experiences impaired ability to perform or complete toileting activities for self

Defining Characteristics
> Unable to
>> Get to commode or toilet
>> Sit on or rise from toilet/commode
>> Carry out proper toilet hygiene
>> Manipulate clothing for toileting
>> Flush toilet or empty commode

Related Factors
> Effects of
>> Aging
>> Chronic illness
>> Cognitive/perceptual impairment
>> Loss of limbs
>> Medications
>> Neuromuscular/musculoskeletal impairment
>> Surgery
>> Trauma
>> Visual impairment
> Lack of
>> Coordination
>> Motivation
>> Self-confidence
> Muscular weakness
> Fatigue
> Pain, discomfort
> Contractures
> Stiffness
> Presence of external devices—IV lines, casts, slings, traction, splints, restraints
> Immobility
> Psychotic states
> Depression
> Knowledge deficit
> Confusion
> Anxiety
> Grieving
> Dependency
> Impaired transfer ability, mobility
> Intolerance to activity
> Decreased strength and endurance

Diagnosis: *Altered Growth and Development*

Definition: The state in which an individual deviates from the norms characteristic of age group

Defining Characteristics
Major
Altered physical growth
Delay or difficulty in performing skills that are typical of age group
Motor
Social
Expressive
Inability to perform self-care or self-control activities appropriate for age
Minor
Flat affect
Decreased responses
Listlessness
Anxiety
Feelings of loneliness, rejection, fear

Related Factors
Effects of physical disability
Environmental and stimulation deficiencies
Inadequate caretaking
Indifference
Inconsistent responsiveness
Multiple caretakers
Prescribed dependence
Separation from significant others

Diagnosis: *Relocation Stress Syndrome*

Definition: Physiological and/or psychological disturbances as a result of transfer from one environment to another

Defining Characteristics
> Major
>> Change in environment/location
>> Anxiety
>> Apprehension
>> Increased confusion (elderly population)
>> Depression
>> Loneliness
> Minor
>> Verbalization of unwillingness to relocate
>> Sleep disturbance
>> Change in eating habits
>> Dependency
>> Gastrointestinal disturbances
>> Increased verbalization of needs
>> Insecurity
>> Lack of trust
>> Restlessness
>> Sad affect
>> Unfavorable comparison of post-/pre-transfer staff
>> Verbalization of being concerned/upset about transfer
>> Vigilance
>> Weight change
>> Withdrawal

Related Factors
> Past, concurrent, and recent losses
> Losses involved with decision to move
> Feeling of powerlessness
> Lack of adequate support system
> Little or no preparation for impending move
> Moderate to high degree of environmental change
> History and types of previous transfers
> Impaired psychosocial health status
> Decreased physical health status

Perceiving
A human response pattern involving the reception of information

 Diagnosis: *Body Image Disturbance*

Definition: The state in which an individual experiences a negative or distorted perception of the body

Defining Characteristics
Either of the following must be present to justify the diagnosis of disturbance in body image:

Verbal response to actual or perceived change in structure and/or function

Nonverbal response to actual or perceived change in structure and/or function

Subjective

Verbalization of

Change in lifestyle

Fear of rejection or of reaction by others

Focus on past strength, function, or appearance

Negative feelings about body

Feelings of helplessness or powerlessness

Preoccupation with change or loss

Emphasis on remaining strengths, heightened achievement

Extension of body boundary to incorporate environmental objects

Refusal to verify actual change or loss

Depersonalization of part or loss by use of impersonal pronouns

Personalization of part or loss by name

Objective

Missing body part

Actual change in structure and/or function

Not looking at or touching body part

Change in ability to estimate spatial relationship of body to environment

Hiding or overexposing body part (intentional or unintentional)

Trauma to nonfunctioning part

Change in social involvement

Related Factors
      Effects of loss of body part(s)
      Effects of loss of body function
      Biophysical
      Cognitive/perceptual
      Cultural or spiritual
      Psychosocial

Diagnosis: *Self-Esteem Disturbance*

Definition: The state in which an individual has negative self-evaluation/feelings about self or self-capabilities, which may be directly or indirectly expressed

Defining Characteristics
Self-negating verbalization
Expresssions of shame/guilt
Evaluates self as unable to deal with events
Rationalizes away/rejects positive feedback and exaggerates
    negative feedback about self
Hesitant to try new things/situations
Denial of problems obvious to others
Projection of blame/responsibility for problems
Rationalizes personal failures
Hypersensitive to a slight or criticism
Grandiosity

Related Factors
To be developed

Diagnosis: *Chronic Low Self-Esteem*

Definition: The state in which an individual has long-standing negative self-evaluation/feelings about self or self-capabilities

Defining Characteristics
Major
Long-standing or chronic:
Self-negating verbalization
Expressions of shame/guilt
Evaluates self as unable to deal with events
Rationalizes away/rejects positive feedback and exaggerates negative feedback about self
Hesitant to try new things/situations

Minor
Frequent lack of success in work or other life events
Overly conforming or dependent on others' opinions
Lack of eye contact
Nonassertive/passive behavior
Indecisive
Excessively seeks reassurance

Related Factors
To be developed

Diagnosis: *Situational Low Self-Esteem*

Definition: The state in which an individual has negative self-evaluation/feelings about self that develop in response to a loss or change in an individual who previously had a positive self-evaluation

Defining Characteristics
Major

Episodic occurrence of negative self-appraisal in response to life events in a person with a previously positive self-evaluation

Verbalization of negative feelings about the self (helplessness, uselessness)

Minor

Self-negating verbalizations

Expressions of shame/guilt

Evaluates self as unable to handle situations/events

Difficulty making decisions

Related Factors
To be developed

Diagnosis: *Personal Identity Disturbance*

Definition: The state in which an individual experiences an inability to distinguish between self and non-self

Defining Characteristics
> To be developed

Related Factors
> Developmental crises
> Role changes
> To be developed

Diagnosis: *Sensory-Perceptual Alterations (Specify):*
Visual, Auditory, Kinesthetic, Gustatory,
Tactile, Olfactory

Definition: A state in which an individual experiences a change in the amount or pattern of in-coming stimuli accompanied by a diminished, exaggerated, distorted, or impaired response to such stimuli

Defining Characteristics

Change in muscle tension
Fatigue
Visual and auditory distortions
Motor incoordination
Alteration in posture
Exaggerated emotional responses
Rapid mood swings
Anxiety
Change in behavior pattern
Apathy
Restlessness
Irritability
Fear
Anger
Depression
Inappropriate responses
Hallucinations
Disordered thought sequence
Bizarre thinking
Daydreaming
Noncompliance
Lack of concentration
Altered conceptualization
Altered communication patterns
Indication of body image alteration
Change in usual response to stimuli
Reported or necessitated change in sensory acuity
Change in problem-solving abilities
Altered abstraction
Disoriented as to time, place, or person

Related Factors

Sleep deprivation
Pain

Chemical alteration
>
> Endogenous (electrolyte imbalance, elevated blood-urea nitrogen, elevated ammonia, hypoxia)
>
> Exogenous (central nervous system stimulants or depressants, mind-altering drugs)

Altered status of sense organs

Effects of neurological disease, trauma, or deficit

Inability to communicate, understand, speak, or respond

Psychological stress or narrowed perceptual fields caused by anxiety

Altered sensory reception, transmission, and/or integration

Socially restricted environment (institutionalization, homebound, aging, chronic illness, dying, infant deprivation, bereaved, stigmatized, mentally ill, mentally retarded, or mentally handicapped)

Environmental factors
>
> Therapeutically restricted environment (isolation, intensive care, bedrest, traction, incubator)

Visual

Defining Characteristics

Headache
Blurring
Spots
Double vision
Excessive tearing
Inflammation
Lack of blink or corneal reflex
Squinting
Holding objects too close or at a distance for viewing
Bumping into objects
Abnormal results of vision testing

Related Factors

Restriction of head/neck motion
Effects of
>
> Aging
> Stress
> Neurological impairment

Failure to use protective eye devices
Improper use of contact lens
Difficulty in adjustment to corrective lens
Persistent visual stimulation

Text continued on following page

Diagnosis: *Sensory-Perceptual Alterations (Specify):*
Visual, Auditory, Kinesthetic, Gustatory,
Tactile, Olfactory (Continued)

Auditory

Defining Characteristics
> Tinnitus
> Abnormal hearing test
> Lack of startle reflex
>> Failure to respond to verbal stimuli
> Cupping of ears
> Inattentiveness
> Withdrawal
> Daydreaming
> Auditory hallucinations
> Inappropriate responses
> Delayed speech or language development

Related Factors
> Effects of aging
> Neurological impairment
> Effects of certain antibiotics
> Excessive ear wax, fluid, or foreign body in ear
> Social isolation
> Stress
> Failure to use protective ear devices
> Continuous exposure to excessive noise
> Psychoses

Kinesthetic

Defining Characteristics
> Falling
> Vertigo
> Stumbling
> Nausea
> Motion sickness
> Motor incoordination
> Alteration in posture
> Inability to sit or stand

Related Factors
> Effects of inner ear inflammation
> Neurological impairment

Side effects of tranquilizers, sedatives, muscle relaxants, or
   antihistamines
Sleep deprivation

Gustatory

Defining Characteristics
Decreased sensitivity to tastes
Decreased appetite
Increased use of seasoning

Related Factors
Inflammation of nasal mucosa
Side effects of certain medications
Aging
Effects of trauma to tongue
Neurological impairment

Tactile

Defining Characteristics
Paresthesias
Hyperesthesias
Anesthesias

Related Factors
Circulatory impairment
Inflammation
Effects of anesthesia
Nutritional deficiencies
Effects of aging
Effects of burns
Neurological impairment
Pain
Persistent tactile stimulation

Olfactory

Defining Characteristics
Decreased sensitivity to smells
Decreased appetite

Related Factors
Inflammation of nasal mucosa
Foreign body in nasal passage
Effects of aging
Neurological impairment

Diagnosis: *Unilateral Neglect*

Definition: The state in which an individual is perceptually unaware of and inattentive to one side of the body

Defining Characteristics
Major
Consistent inattention to stimuli on affected side
Minor
Does not look toward affected side
Leaves food on plate on the affected side
Inadequate self-care, positioning, and/or safety precautions in regard to affected side

Related Factors
Effects of disturbed perceptual abilities, e.g.,
Hemianopsia
One-sided blindness
Effects of neurological illness or trauma

Diagnosis: *Hopelessness*

Definition: The subjective state in which an individual sees limited or no alternatives or personal choices available and is unable to mobilize energy on own behalf

Defining Characteristics
> Major
>> Passivity
>> Decreased verbalization
>> Verbal cues (despondent content, "I can't," sighing)
> Minor
>> Increased or decreased sleep
>> Decreased appetite
>> Closing eyes
>> Turning away from speaker
>> Lack of involvement in care or passively allowing care
>> Shrugging in response to speaker
>> Decreased response to stimuli
>> Lack of initiative
>> Flat affect

Related Factors
> Chronic pain
> Effects of
>> Deteriorating physiological condition
>> Long-term stress
>> Abandonment
>> Role disruption
>> Loss of significant other
> Grieving
> Depression
> Prolonged activity restriction creating isolation
> Lost belief in religious values

Diagnosis: *Powerlessness*

Definition: The state in which an individual experiences the perception that one's own actions will not significantly affect an outcome or a perceived lack of control over a current situation or immediate happening

Defining Characteristics
>Severe
>>Verbal expressions of
>>>Having no control or influence over situation
>>>Having no control or influence over outcome
>>>Having no control over self-care
>>Depression over physical deterioration that occurs despite patient's compliance with regimen
>>Apathy
>>Expressions of uncertainty about fluctuating energy levels
>>Passivity
>Moderate
>>Nonparticipation in care or decision making when opportunities are provided
>>Expressions of dissatisfaction and frustration over inability to perform tasks and/or activities
>>No attempt to monitor progress
>>Expressions of doubt about self-worth or role performance
>>Reluctance to express true feelings
>>Fearing alienation from caregivers
>>Passivity
>>Inability to seek information regarding care
>>Dependence on others that may result in
>>>Irritability
>>>Resentment
>>>Anger
>>>Guilt
>>Does not defend self-care practices when challenged

Related Factors
>Immobility
>Difficulty in performing self-care
>Illness-related regimen
>Social isolation

Low self-esteem
Cultural role
Communication barriers
Loss of financial independence
Lifestyle of helplessness
Interpersonal interactions
Lack of knowledge or skills
Health care environment

Knowing

A human response pattern involving meaning associated with information

 Diagnosis: *Knowledge Deficit (Specify)*

Definition: The state in which an individual lacks specific knowledge or skills that affect ability to maintain health

Defining Characteristics

Verbalizes the problem
Inaccurate
    Follow-through of instruction
    Use of health-related vocabulary
    Performance of test
Expresses inaccurate perception of problem
Inability to explain therapeutic regimen or describe personal
    health status
Repeatedly requests information
Failure to seek help or follow therapeutic regimen
Inappropriate or exaggerated behaviors, e.g., hysteria,
    hostility, apathy, agitation, depression
Failure to take medication

Related Factors

Effects of
    Aging
    Sensory deficits
    Language barrier
    Cognitive limitations
Information misinterpretation
Unfamiliarity with information resources
Lack of
    Interest in learning
    Exposure
    Recall
Denial
Substance abuse
Self-destructive patterns
Inadequate economic resources

Diagnosis: *Altered Thought Processes*

Definition: The state in which the individual experiences a disruption in cognitive operations and activities

Defining Characteristics
Agitation or depressed behavior
Altered sleep patterns
Inappropriate affect or social behavior
Non–reality-based thinking
Fabrication
Confabulations
Egocentricity
Obsessions
Cognitive dissonance
Hyper-/hypovigilance
Nonsensical speech
Inability to perceive and/or repeat message clearly
Inaccurate interpretation of environment
Memory deficits
Distractibility
Disorientation as to time, place, person
Impaired ability to make decisions, problem solve, reason,
   abstract, conceptualize, calculate
Delusions or hallucinations
Ideas of reference
Decreased response to simple requests

Related Factors
Effects of
   Aging
   Medications
      Sedatives
      Narcotics
      Anesthetics
   Sleep deprivation
   Psychological conflicts
   Loss of memory
   Depression
   Stress
   Anxiety
   Social isolation
   Emotional trauma
   Fear of the unknown

Text continued on following page

Diagnosis: *Altered Thought Processes (Continued)*

Negative reactions from others
Actual loss of:
   Control
   Familiar objects
   Routine surroundings
   Income
   Significant other
Limited attention span
Impaired judgment
Sensory overload or deprivation
Exposure to unfamiliar environment

Feeling

A human response pattern involving the subjective awareness of information

 Diagnosis: *Pain*

Definition: The state in which an individual experiences and reports the presence of severe discomfort or an uncomfortable sensation

Defining Characteristics

    Subjective

        Communication (verbal or coded) of pain descriptors

    Objective

        Guarding behavior, protective

        Self-focusing

        Narrowed focus

            Altered time perception

            Withdrawal from social contact

            Impaired thought process

    Distraction behavior

        Moaning

        Crying

        Pacing

        Seeking out other people and/or activities

        Restlessness

    Clutching of painful area

    Trembling

    Facial mask of pain

        Eyes lack luster

        "Beaten" look

        Fixed or scattered movement

        Grimace

    Changes in posture or gait

    Positive response to palpation

    Withdrawal reflex

    Changes in muscle tone(may range from listless to rigid)

    Autonomic responses (not seen in chronic stable pain)

        Increased blood pressure, pulse, respirations

        Diaphoresis

        Dilated pupils

    Reports of pain

Text continued on following page

Diagnosis: *Pain (Continued)*

Related Factors
>Inflammation
>Muscle spasm
>Effects of surgery or trauma
>Immobility
>Obstructive processes
>Pressure points
>Infectious process
>Experiences during diagnostic tests
>Overactivity
>Injury agents
>>Biological
>>Chemical
>>Physical
>>Psychological

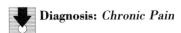 **Diagnosis:** *Chronic Pain*

Definition: The state in which an individual experiences pain that continues for more than 6 months

Defining Characteristics
>Major
>>Verbal report or observed evidence of pain experienced for more than 6 months
>
>Minor
>>Facial masks of pain
>>Anorexia
>>Weight changes
>>Changes in sleep patterns
>>Insomnia
>>Guarded movement
>>Depression
>>Personality changes
>>Irritability
>>Fear of reinjury
>>Altered ability to continue previous activities
>>Physical and social withdrawal

Related Factors
>Effects of chronic or terminal illness
>Muscle spasm
>Inflammation
>Chronic psychosocial disability

Diagnosis: *Dysfunctional Grieving*

Definition: The state in which an individual experiences an exaggerated response to an actual or potential loss of person, relationship, object, or functional abilities

Defining Characteristics
> Verbal expression of distress at loss
> Expression of unresolved issues
> Crying
> Weight loss
> Amenorrhea
> Changes in
>> Sleep patterns
>> Activity
>> Eating patterns
>> Dream patterns
>> Libido
> Feelings of
>> Anger
>> Guilt
>> Worthlessness
>> Denial
>> Sadness
>> Sorrow
> Decreased interest in personal appearance
> Interference with life functioning
> Reliving of past experiences
> Difficulty in expressing loss
> Alterations in concentration and/or pursuit of tasks
> Developmental regression
> Hyperactivity
> Fear of future
> Absence of emotion
> Suicidal thoughts
> Social withdrawal
> Labile affect

Related Factors
> Effects of actual or perceived loss of significant other, health
> or social status, or valued object
>> People
>> Possessions
>> Job status

Home
Ideals
Parts and processes of the body
Absence of anticipatory grieving
Thwarted grieving in response to a loss
Effects of multiple losses or crises
Lack of resolution of previous grieving response
Ambivalent feelings toward loss
Changes in lifestyle
Decreased support system

Diagnosis: *Anticipatory Grieving*

Definition: The state in which an individual experiences responses to an actual or perceived loss of a person, relationship, object, or functional abilities before the loss occurs

Defining Characteristics
> Altered affect
> Anger
> Guilt
> Sorrow
> Choked feelings
> Expressed distress at potential loss
> Altered libido
> Denial of potential loss
> Changes in activity levels, sleeping, or eating habits
> Crying
> Altered communication patterns

Related Factors
> Effects of actual or potential loss of significant other, health status, social status, or valued object

High-Risk Diagnosis: *High Risk for Violence: Self-Directed or Directed at Others*

Definition: The state in which an individual experiences behaviors that can be physically harmful to self or others

Risk Factors

 Substance abuse or withdrawal
 Toxic reaction to medication
 Explosive, impulsive, immature personality
 Paranoia
 Panic states
 Rage reactions
 Manic excitement
 Loneliness
 Perceived threat to self-esteem
 Response to catastrophic event
 Suicidal behavior
 Antisocial characteristics
 Dysfunctional communication patterns
 Change in mental or physical health status
 Feelings of alienation
 Catatonic excitement
 Physical, sexual, or psychological abuse (battered women, children, or elderly)
 Manipulative behavior
 Developmental crisis
 Lack of support systems
 Actual or potential loss of significant other
 Social isolation
 Significant change in lifestyle
 Effects of
  Organic brain syndrome
  Temporal lobe epilepsy

High-Risk Diagnosis: *High Risk for Self-Mutilation*

Definition: A state in which an individual is at high risk for performing an act on the self to injure, not kill, which produces tissue damage and tension relief

Risk Factors

Groups at risk

Clients with borderline personality disorder, especially females 16–25 years of age

Clients in psychotic state—frequently males in young adulthood

Emotionally disturbed and/or battered children

Mentally retarded and autistic children

Clients with a history of self-injury

History of physical, emotional, or sexual abuse

Inability to cope with increased psychological/physiological tension in a healthy manner

Feelings of depression, rejection, self-hatred, separation anxiety, guilt, and depersonalization

Fluctuating emotions

Command hallucinations

Need for sensory stimuli

Parental emotional deprivation

Dysfunctional family

Diagnosis: *Post-Trauma Response*

Definition: The state in which an individual experiences a sustained painful response to an overwhelming traumatic event

Defining Characteristics
 Major
  Re-experiencing traumatic event through
   Flashbacks
   Intrusive thoughts
   Repetitive dreams or nightmares
   Excessive verbalization of traumatic event, verbalization of survival guilt or guilt about behavior required for survival

 Minor
  Psychic/emotional numbness
   Impaired interpretation of reality
   Confusion
   Dissociation or amnesia
   Vagueness about traumatic event
   Constricted affect
  Altered lifestyle
   Substance abuse
   Suicide attempt or other acting-out behavior
   Difficulty with interpersonal relationships
   Development of phobia regarding trauma
   Decreased impulse control/irritability and explosiveness

Related Factors
 Effects of
  Disasters
  Wars
  Epidemics
  Rape
  Assault
  Torture
  Catastrophic illness or accident

Diagnosis: *Rape-Trauma Syndrome*

Definition: Forced, violent sexual penetration against the victim's will and consent. The trauma syndrome that results from this attack or attempted attack includes an acute phase of disorganization of the victim's lifestyle and a long-term reorganization of lifestyle.

Defining Characteristics
    Acute phase
        Emotional reactions
            Anger
            Crying
            Overcontrol
            Panic
            Denial
            Revenge
            Self-blame
            Emotional shock
            Embarrassment
            Fear of being alone
            Humiliation
            Fear of physical violence and death
            Desire for revenge
            Change in sexual behavior
            Mistrust of opposite sex
        Multiple physical symptoms
            Muscle tension
            Pain
            Sleep pattern disturbance
            Gastrointestinal irritability
            Genitourinary discomfort
    Long-term phase
        Mentally reliving rape
        Ambivalence about own sexuality
        Seeking family or social network support
        Changes in lifestyle
            Changes in residence
            Dealing with repetitive nightmares and phobias
        Depression
        Anxiety
        Loss of self-confidence

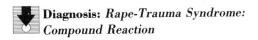

Diagnosis: *Rape-Trauma Syndrome:*
Compound Reaction

Definition: Forced, violent sexual penetration against the victim's will and consent. The trauma syndrome that results from this attack or attempted attack includes an acute phase of disorganization of the victim's lifestyle and a long-term reorganization of lifestyle

Defining Characteristics
　　Acute phase
　　　　Emotional reactions
　　　　　　Anger
　　　　　　Embarrrassment
　　　　　　Fear of physical violence and death
　　　　　　Humiliation
　　　　　　Revenge
　　　　　　Self-blame
　　　　Multiple physical symptoms
　　　　　　Gastrointestinal irritability
　　　　　　Genitourinary discomfort
　　　　　　Muscle tension
　　　　　　Sleep pattern disturbance
　　　　Reactivated symptoms of previous conditions
　　　　　　Physical illness
　　　　　　Psychiatric illness
　　　　Reliance on alcohol or drugs
　　Long-term phase
　　　　Change in lifestyle
　　　　　　Change in residence
　　　　　　Dealing with repetitive nightmares and phobias
　　　　　　Seeking family support
　　　　　　Seeking social network support

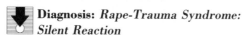 **Diagnosis:** *Rape-Trauma Syndrome:*
Silent Reaction

Definition: Forced, violent sexual penetration against the victim's will and consent. The trauma syndrome that results from this attack or attempted attack includes an acute phase of disorganization of the victim's lifestyle and a long-term reorganization of lifestyle

Defining Characteristics

    Abrupt changes in relationships with opposite sex
    Increase in nightmares
    Increasing anxiety during interviews, e.g., blocking of associations, long periods of silence, minor stuttering, physical distress
    Marked changes in sexual behavior
    No verbalization of the occurrence of rape
    Sudden onset of phobic reactions

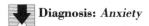 **Diagnosis:** *Anxiety*

Definition: The state in which an individual experiences a vague uneasy feeling, the source of which is often nonspecific or unknown

Defining Characteristics
    Subjective
        Increased tension
        Apprehension
        Painful and persistent increased helplessness
        Uncertainty
        Fearfulness
        Scared
        Regretful
        Overexcited
        Rattled
        Distressed
        Jittery
        Feelings of inadequacy
        Shakiness
        Fear of unspecified consequences
        Expressed concerns regarding change in life events
        Worried
        Anxious
    Objective
        Sympathetic stimulation
            Cardiovascular excitation
            Superficial vasoconstriction
            Pupil dilation
            Increased perspiration
        Restlessness
        Insomnia
        Glancing about
        Lack of eye contact
        Trembling/hand tremors
        Extraneous movement
            Foot shuffling
            Hand/arm movements
        Facial tension
        Voice quivering
        Focus on self
        Increased wariness

Related Factors
    Loss of possessions
    Effects of actual or perceived loss of significant others
Text continued on following page

Diagnosis: *Anxiety (Continued)*

Threat to or change in health status, socioeconomic status, relationships, role functioning, support systems, environment, self-concept, or interaction patterns
Situational and maturational crises
Unmet needs
Threat of death
Unconscious conflict about essential values and goals of life
Lack of knowledge
Loss of control
Feelings of failure
Disruptive family life
Interpersonal transmission and contagion
Threat to self-concept

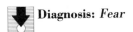 **Diagnosis:** *Fear*

Definition: The state in which the individual experiences feelings of dread related to an identifiable source perceived as dangerous

Defining Characteristics
    Ability to identify object of fear
    Sympathetic stimulation
        Cardiovascular excitation
        Superficial vasoconstriction
        Increased blood pressure, pulse, and respirations
    Wide-eyed appearance
    Crying
    Voice tremors
    Diaphoresis
    Urinary frequency
    Regressive behavior, pacing
    Withdrawing
    Insomnia
    Terror
    Panic
    Apprehension
    Aggression
    Increased alertness
    Decreased self-assurance
    Increased questioning/verbalization
    Feelings of loss of control

Related Factors
    Sensory impairment, deprivation, or overload
    Pain
    Effects of loss of body part or function
    Effects of chronic disabling illness
    Language barrier
    Threat of death, actual or perceived
    Anticipation of events posing a threat to self-esteem
    Phobias
    Feelings of failure
    Knowledge deficit
    Learned response, conditioning
    Loss of significant other
    Separation from support system

Care Planning: Nursing Diagnoses and Outcomes

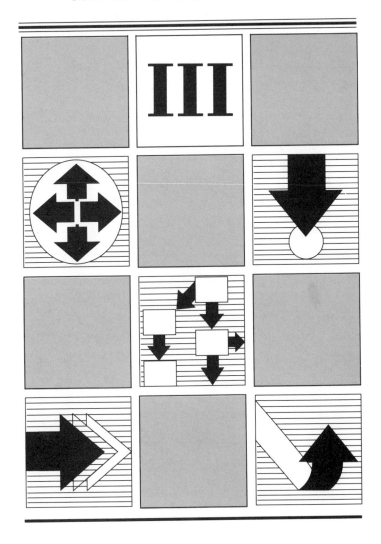

This section includes common nursing diagnoses and sample client outcomes for 34 high-frequency medical diagnoses. When writing care plans, readers can refer to this section for assistance in formulating correctly stated nursing diagnoses and outcomes. The diagnoses and outcomes have been incorporated under the major diagnostic categories of the Diagnostic Related Grouping (DRG) system. Table 3–1 illustrates this grouping. In addition, an alphabetized list of the common medical diagnoses can be found on page 189.

The following is a list of frequently used abbreviations and their definitions:

ABG—arterial blood gases

ADL—activities of daily living

A/P—apical pulse

B/P—blood pressure

BSE—breast self-examination

CVP—central venous pressure

D/D—diseases and/or disorders

ET—endotracheal tube

H&H—hemoglobin and hematocrit

I&O—intake and output

L/R—left/right

MVA—motor vehicle accident

N/G—nasogastric

NPO—nothing by mouth

N/V— nausea and vomiting

P—pulse

PTT—partial thromboplastin time

R—respirations

ROM—range of motion

R/T—related to

WBC—white blood count

WNL—within normal limits

2°—secondary to

■ **Table 3–1. Major Diagnostic Categories of the DRG System and High-Frequency Medical Diagnoses**

Major Diagnostic Category	Disease/Disorder
1. D/D of nervous system	Cerebrovascular accident Transient ischemic attack
4. D/D of the respiratory system	Asthma Chronic obstructive pulmonary disease Pneumonia Pulmonary embolism Respiratory failure

Table continued on following page

Major Diagnostic Category	Disease/Disorder
	Thoracic surgery Tuberculosis
5. D/D of the circulatory system	Angina Cardiac arrhythmia Cardiac catheterization Congestive heart failure Myocardial infarction Pacemaker Percutaneous transluminal coronary angioplasty
6. D/D of the digestive system	Colostomy Gastroenteritis Gastrointestinal bleeding Gastric ulcer
7. D/D of the hepatobiliary system	Cholecystitis/cholelithiasis
8. D/D of the musculoskeletal system	Back pain Hip fracture Joint procedures
9. D/D of the skin, subcutaneous tissue, breast	Mastectomy
10. Endocrine, nutritional, metabolic diseases	Diabetes
11. D/D of the kidney and urinary tract	Transurethral resection of the prostate Urinary tract infection
14. Pregnancy, childbirth, and puerperium	Cesarean birth Normal vaginal delivery
15. Newborns and other neonates with conditions originating in the perinatal period	High-risk newborn Normal newborn
17. Myeloproliferative D/D, poorly differentiated neoplasms	Terminal cancer
18. Infectious and parasitic diseases	Acquired immune deficiency syndrome (AIDS) Septicemia
19. Mental D/D	Alzheimer's disease Depression Psychoses
20. Substance use and substance-induced organic mental disorders	Substance abuse
Miscellaneous	Preoperative Postoperative

High-Frequency Medical Diagnoses

▌ D/D of the Nervous System

 Cerebrovascular Accident

Nursing Diagnosis	Client Outcomes
Altered cerebral tissue perfusion R/T effects of decreased/absent blood flow	Throughout hospitalization, no evidence of deteriorating neurological signs
High risk for aspiration R/T retained secretions, effects of L/R-sided weakness, impaired swallowing, impaired gag reflex	Throughout hospitalization, no evidence of aspiration
Impaired verbal communication R/T dysarthria, dysphagia, aphasia	During hospitalization, utilizes alternative methods to communicate
High risk for impaired skin integrity R/T prolonged immobility, incontinence, altered nutritional status	No evidence of skin breakdown over bony prominences throughout hospitalization
Impaired physical mobility R/T effects of L/R-sided weakness, hemiplegia, decreased level of consciousness	Prior to discharge, full ROM in all extremities
Feeding self-care deficit R/T impaired physical mobility, visual impairments	Prior to discharge, feeds self using adaptive equipment
Unilateral neglect (L/R side) R/T effects of visual changes	Demonstrates attention to affected side during hospitalization
Reflex incontinence R/T loss of bladder tone, sphincter control	Voids at least ___ ml q ___ Experiences decreased episodes of incontinence by time of discharge
Colonic constipation R/T decreased mobility, decreased oral intake, inability to verbalize needs	Prior to discharge, resumes normal elimination pattern q ___

Nursing Diagnosis	Client Outcomes
Altered nutrition: less than body requirements R/T dysphagia, inability to feed self	Weight loss no greater than ___ lb during hospitalization
High risk for disuse syndrome R/T prolonged immobility	No evidence of complications of immobility during hospitalization
Fear R/T uncertain diagnosis, effects of disease on lifestyle	Demonstrates decreased fear within 48 hours
Altered thought processes: confusion R/T cerebral ischemia	When reoriented, correctly identifies person, place, and time
Ineffective denial R/T perceived changes in lifestyle	Prior to discharge: Realistically describes impact of disease. Identifies positive coping strategies to manage lifestyle change
Impaired social interaction R/T decreased mobility, impaired communication	Prior to discharge: Communicates feelings to person of choice. Identifies alternatives to maintain social contacts
Impaired adjustment R/T awareness of physical limitations, change in body image and lifestyle	Prior to discharge, identifies strategies and support systems to assist with adjustment
High risk for trauma R/T decreased mobility, weakness, perceptual impairment	During hospitalization, no evidence of accident or injury
Impaired home maintenance management R/T sensorimotor deficits	Prior to discharge, identifies alternative resources for home maintenance

Text continued on following page

Cerebrovascular Accident *Continued*

Nursing Diagnosis	Client Outcomes
Knowledge deficit (disease process, activity limitations, medication therapy, follow-up care)	Prior to discharge, patient/family: Defines disease process Names activity limitations Identifies action, dosage, and major side effects of prescribed medications Explains the need for and describes plans for follow-up care

**Transient Ischemic Attack
(Acute Requiring Hospitalization)**

Nursing Diagnosis	Client Outcomes
Fear R/T uncertainty of diagnosis and outcome, effects of disease on lifestyle	Verbalizes decreased fear within ___.
Altered protection R/T effects of anticoagulation therapy	Throughout period of anticoagulation: Coagulation studies within desired limits No evidence of bleeding
Altered cerebral tissue perfusion R/T effects of transient interruption of cerebral blood flow	No evidence of deterioration of neurological signs throughout hospitalization
Altered visual sensory-perception R/T effects of decreased cerebral oxygenation	Adjusts environment to compensate for temporary vision loss
Ineffective denial R/T perceived changes in lifestyle secondary to disease process	Prior to discharge: Acknowledges presence of disease Realistically describes impact of disease
Impaired physical mobility R/T effects of temporary R/L-sided weakness	Prior to discharge, ambulates and transfers independently or with assistance
High risk for altered thought processes R/T effects of cerebral ischemia	Throughout hospitalization, maintains pre-episode level of orientation
Knowledge deficit (disease process, risk factors, diet, medications, follow-up care)	Defines disease process Identifies own risk factors Selects appropriate foods from menu Explains action, dosage and major side effects of prescribed medications Describes the importance of and states plans for follow-up care

D/D of Respiratory System

 Asthma

Nursing Diagnosis	Client Outcomes
Ineffective airway clearance R/T retained secretions, narrow airways	No evidence of respiratory distress during hospitalization
Ineffective breathing pattern R/T fatigue, anxiety	Respiratory rate, rhythm, and depth WNL for client within _____ hours
Inability to sustain spontaneous ventilation R/T respiratory muscle fatigue	Breathes without mechanical assistance throughout hospitalization
Pain R/T muscle spasm, coughing	Expresses comfort within 45 minutes after initiation of comfort measures
Fatigue R/T hypoxia, increased energy requirements for ADL	Participates in ADL without reports of fatigue prior to discharge
Sleep-pattern disturbance R/T anxiety, dyspnea, hospital routine	Experiences at least 4 hours of uninterrupted sleep twice within 24 hours
Impaired verbal communication R/T dyspnea	Within __ hours communicates needs using alternative methods
Anxiety R/T dyspnea, fear of death, suffocation	Verbalizes decreasing anxiety within 24 hours
Ineffective individual coping R/T fear of recurrence, changes in lifestyle, inadequate support systems	Prior to discharge, identifies positive strategies to manage effects of disease
Powerlessness R/T effects of recurrent disease, lifestyle restrictions	Verbalizes increased feelings of control prior to discharge

Nursing Diagnosis	Client Outcomes
Knowledge deficit (disease process, precipitating factors, diet, activity, medications, follow-up care)	Prior to discharge, client/ family: Explains disease process and precipitating factors Selects appropriate foods from menu Describes activity limitations, recommended exercises Names action, dosage, and major side effects of prescribed medications Explains the need for and describes plans for follow-up care

Chronic Obstructive Pulmonary Disease (COPD, Acute Episode Requiring Hospitalization)

Nursing Diagnosis	Client Outcomes
Activity intolerance R/T dyspnea, fatigue	B/P, P, and R WNL for client during periods of activity
Fatigue R/T hypoxia, increased energy requirements for ADL	Participates in ADL without reports of fatigue prior to discharge
Impaired verbal communication R/T dyspnea, fatigue	Utilizes alternative form of communication when dyspneic
Constipation R/T immobility, decreased fluid intake	Resumes normal elimination pattern q___ prior to discharge
High risk for infection R/T retained viscous secretions	No evidence of respiratory infection throughout hospitalization
Altered nutrition: less than body requirements R/T anorexia, dyspnea	Weight loss no greater than ___ lb during hospitalization
Altered oral mucous membranes: dryness R/T mouth breathing, oxygen therapy	Moist mucous membranes q shift
High risk for aspiration R/T excessive/viscous secretions	No evidence of aspiration q shift
Impaired gas exchange R/T CO_2 retention, retained pulmonary secretions	ABG WNL for client within ___ days. Breath sounds present bilaterally q shift
Feeding self-care deficit R/T dyspnea, fatigue	Throughout hospitalization, feeds self independently or with assistance consistent with abilities
High risk for impaired skin integrity R/T prolonged immobility, decreased tissue perfusion	During hospitalization, no evidence of skin breakdown over bony prominences
Sleep pattern disturbance R/T sensory overload, nocturnal dyspnea, hospital routine	Experiences at least 3 hours of uninterrupted sleep three times q 24 hours

Nursing Diagnosis	Client Outcomes
Anxiety R/T breathlessness, fear of death	Verbalizes decreased anxiety within __ hours
Impaired adjustment R/T inability to accept necessary lifestyle modifications	Prior to discharge: Verbalizes feelings about lifestyle changes Expresses ability to adapt to needed modifications
Ineffective management of therapeutic regimen (individual) R/T previous unsuccessful experience with prescribed regimen	Verbalizes intent to follow recommended treatment regimen before discharge
Powerlessness R/T lifestyle restrictions, prognosis	Prior to discharge, expresses feelings of increased control over lifestyle
Altered thought processes: confusion R/T decreased cerebral perfusion	Alert and oriented to person, place, and time q shift
Impaired home maintenance management R/T activity limitations secondary to disease process	Prior to discharge, identifies alternatives for home maintenance management
Caregiver role strain R/T age, lack of preparation for caregiver role	Caregiver verbalizes strategies to deal with identified client care problems
Knowledge deficit (disease process, planned therapy, activity, exercise, medications, follow-up care)	Prior to discharge, client/family: Describes disease process (COPD) Discusses prescribed treatment regimen Explains activity limitations Identifies need for exercise and demonstrates those prescribed Names action, dosage, and major side effects of prescribed medications Explains need for and describes plans for follow-up care

Pneumonia

Nursing Diagnosis	Client Outcomes
Ineffective breathing pattern R/T persistent pain, fatigue	Throughout hospitalization, respiratory rate, rhythm, and depth WNL for patient
Ineffective airway clearance R/T dehydration, viscous secretions	Throughout hospitalization, no evidence of respiratory distress
	Coughs and expectorates thinned secretions q ___
Fluid volume deficit R/T decreased fluid intake, diaphoresis, hyperthermia	Consumes at least ___ ml of fluid q 24 hours
Hyperthermia R/T dehydration, decreased fluid intake	Temperature below 101°F within 24 hours
Altered nutrition: less than body requirements R/T anorexia, dyspnea, increased metabolism	Consumes at least ___ calories q 24 hours
Pain R/T pleuritic inflammation, persistent cough	Verbalizes comfort within minutes after initiation of comfort measure
Sleep pattern disturbance R/T pain, excessive coughing, hospital routine	Within 48 hours, experiences at least 4 hours of uninterrupted sleep q 24 hours
Anxiety R/T dyspnea, pleuritic pain	Within 48 hours, verbalizes decreased anxiety
Knowledge deficit (activity limitation, prescribed medications)	Before discharge: Identifies own activity limitations
	Names action, dosage, and major side effects of prescribed medications

Pulmonary Embolism

Nursing Diagnosis	Client Outcomes
Impaired gas exchange R/T obstructive process	ABG WNL within 24 hours
Impaired physical mobility R/T reluctance to move, fear of dislodgment of clot	Participates in ADL within prescribed limitations throughout hospitalization
Bathing self-care deficit R/T dyspnea, pain, decreased mobility, fear	Bathes self consistent with abilities and activity restrictions throughout hospitalization
Pain R/T obstructive process	Expresses comfort within ___ minutes after initiation of comfort measure
High risk for fluid volume deficit R/T hemorrhage secondary to anticoagulant, thrombolytic therapy	No evidence of unusual bleeding during drug therapy
Fatigue R/T hypoxia, increased energy requirements for ADL	Verbalizes decreased fatigue within ___
Sleep pattern disturbance R/T anxiety, hospital routines	Throughout hospitalization sleeps at least ___ uninterrupted hours q 24 hours
Fear R/T dyspnea, chest pain, possibility of recurrence	Prior to discharge, verbalizes decreased fearfulness
Knowledge deficit (disease process, anticoagulant therapy, need for follow-up care)	Prior to discharge: Identifies causes of thrombus formation Verbalizes rationale for dosage and side effects of anticoagulants States need for and describes plan for follow-up care

Acute Respiratory Failure

Nursing Diagnosis	Client Outcomes
Impaired gas exchange R/T hypoxia 2° effects of decreased functional lung tissue, interstitial/alveolar edema	Within ___: No evidence of respiratory distress Respiratory rate, pattern, depth WNL for client Breath sounds present bilaterally q shift ABGs within desired limits (specify) Pulmonary function studies WNL for client Chest x-ray film clear

For Mechanically Ventilated Clients

Nursing Diagnosis	Client Outcomes
Fear R/T threat of death, inability to breathe, malfunction of ventilator, inability to communicate	Verbalizes decreased fear within ___ using established alternative communication system
High risk for ineffective airway clearance R/T effects of artificial airway and mechanical ventilation	While artificial airway in place: Patent airway Clear breath sounds No signs/symptoms of respiratory distress
High risk for ineffective breathing patterns R/T anxiety/fear 2° mechanical ventilation	Within ___ : Respiratory rate within prescribed parameters ___ breaths/min (synchronized with ventilator) High-pressure alarms silent
High risk for impaired tissue integrity R/T pressure 2° cuffed airway	While airway in place: No evidence of tracheal/esophageal erosion or fistula
High risk for impaired skin integrity R/T pressure 2° endotracheal tube (ET) placement	While tube in place: No evidence of skin breakdown on face
High risk for impaired oral mucous membranes R/T trauma 2° ET/trach placement and NPO status	While intubated, no evidence of ulcerated oral mucous membranes

Nursing Diagnosis	Client Outcomes
High risk for infection R/T effects of invasive ET/trach placement	Throughout hospitalization, no evidence of local/systemic infection
High risk for aspiration R/T hazards associated with artificial airway	No evidence of aspiration while ET/trach in place
Altered nutrition: less than body requirements R/T decreased oral intake 2° ET/trach placement	Weight loss no greater than ___ lb within ___
High risk for disuse syndrome R/T prolonged immobility, 2° mechanical ventilation, decreased level of consciousness	No evidence of complications associated with immobility
Activity intolerance R/T increased oxygen demand, fatigue	Performs ADL without fatigue prior to discharge
Impaired verbal communication R/T effects of artificial airway placement	Within ___, establishes and utilizes alternative means of communication
High risk for altered thought processes R/T sleep deprivation 2° mechanical ventilation, sensory overload, perceived loss of control	While on mechanical ventilation, no evidence of restlessness, anxiety, disorientation, paranoia

Weaning the Ventilated Client

Dysfunctional ventilatory weaning response R/T effects of prolonged mechanical ventilation, fear of withdrawal of ventilator, environmental factors	Throughout weaning process: Verbalizes comfort and adequacy of ventilation B/P, P, and R WNL for client ABG WNL for client
High risk for impaired gas exchange R/T hypo-/hyperventilation 2° weaning process	Within ___: ABGs within desired limits (specify) ___ Respiratory rate ___ per minute Tidal volume ___ ml/kg

Text continued on following page

Acute Respiratory Failure *Continued*

Nursing Diagnosis	Client Outcomes *Continued*
Fear R/T perceived threat of death, inability to breathe 2° weaning process	During weaning process: Communicates fears to nurse or person of choice Communicates decreased fear within ___

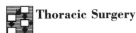 **Thoracic Surgery**

Nursing Diagnosis	Client Outcomes
Pain R/T effects of surgery, presence of chest tube	Expresses comfort within ___ minutes after initiation of comfort measure(s)
High risk for aspiration R/T retained copious secretions	Throughout hospitalization, no evidence of aspiration
High risk for infection R/T effects of surgery	No evidence of infection throughout hospitalization
Ineffective airway clearance R/T retained secretions, reluctance to cough, incisional pain	Within 48 hours: No evidence of respiratory distress; Breath sounds present bilaterally; ABG WNL for client
High risk for injury R/T clotting in chest tube, tubing disconnection, air leak	While chest tube in place: Free flow of blood/air from pleural cavity; Intact drainage system; No evidence of air leak
Impaired physical mobility: L/R arm R/T pain, fear of movement	By time of discharge, full ROM ___ arm/shoulder
Activity intolerance R/T pain, fatigue	Throughout hospitalization, gradually increases participation in ADL according to ability
Altered nutrition: less than body requirements R/T increased metabolic requirements, decreased oral intake	Consumes at least ___ calories/day; Weight loss no greater than ___ lb during hospitalization
Fear R/T outcome of surgery, postoperative pain, chest tube	Prior to discharge, verbalizes decreased fear
Knowledge deficit (post discharge care)	Prior to discharge: Demonstrates wound care; Verbalizes activity limitations; States symptoms to report to physician

Tuberculosis

Nursing Diagnosis	Client Outcomes
Ineffective management of therapeutic regimen R/T lack of understanding of importance of drug therapy, follow-up care, lack of financial resources	Takes medication as ordered Makes and keeps follow-up appointments
Ineffective airway clearance R/T retained secretions, effects of infectious process	Throughout hospitalization, coughs and expectorates secretions
Situational low self-esteem R/T stigma associated with disease	Verbalizes positive feelings about self prior and ability to manage interpersonal issues prior to discharge
Fear R/T effects of disease process, potential complications of therapy	Verbalizes decreased fear within _____
Altered protection R/T effects of therapy, immunosupression, coexisting disease (human immunodeficiency virus [HIV], diabetes)	Throughout treatment regimen, no evidence of complications of therapy, secondary infection
High risk for infection (family, social contacts) R/T exposure to infected client, decreased health status, risk factors	No evidence of tuberculosis in family or social contacts
Social isolation R/T fear of transmission to others, stigma associated with disease	Interacts with family, social contacts at least once daily prior to discharge
Altered nutrition: less than body requirements R/T effects of disease process, anorexia secondary to medication therapy	Weight loss no greater than ___ lb within _____

Nursing Diagnosis	Client Outcomes
Knowledge deficit (disease process, transmission, infection control measures, medication, support systems, follow-up care)	Prior to discharge: Describes disease process, methods of transmission, and infection control measures Names action, dosage, and major side effects of prescribed medications Identifies medical, social, and financial support systems Explains the need for and describes plans for follow-up care

D/D of the Circulatory System

 Angina

Nursing Diagnosis	Client Outcomes
Pain R/T decreased myocardial oxygen supply	Expresses comfort within ___ minutes after initiation of comfort measures
Activity intolerance R/T fear of recurrent chest pain	B/P, P, and R do not exceed recommended limits during activity
Altered sexuality patterns R/T fear of recurrent chest pain	Before discharge: Discusses feelings with person of choice Identifies limitations in sexual activity and describes alternatives
Sleep pattern disturbances R/T anxiety, hospital routines, preoccupation with potential limitations	Within 24 hours, experiences at least 4 hours of uninterrupted sleep twice daily
Altered cardiopulmonary tissue perfusion R/T obstructive process, coronary artery spasm	Throughout hospitalization, verbalizes decreased frequency of chest pain
Ineffective denial R/T perceived lifestyle/role changes	Prior to discharge: States realistic description of change in lifestyle/role Identifies positive strategies to deal with actual lifestyle/role changes
Fear R/T possibility of death, severe pain	Within hours, verbalizes decreased fearfulness
Situational low self-esteem R/T role change secondary to perceived physical limitations	Prior to discharge: Identifies actual physical limitations Verbalizes positive feelings about own abilities

Nursing Diagnosis	Client Outcomes
Altered thought processes: confusion R/T sensory overload and lack of sleep	When reoriented, correctly identifies person, place, and time
Altered health maintenance R/T denial of disease and presence of risk factors	Prior to discharge: Verbalizes disease process by name Identifies own risk factors and methods of decreasing or eliminating
Impaired home maintenance management R/T fear of recurrent chest pain	Prior to discharge, lists alternatives for providing home maintenance
Knowledge deficit (risk factors, low-fat/low-cholesterol diet, medications, follow-up care)	Before discharge: Identifies own risk factors and names methods of management Selects appropriate foods from menu Names actions, dosage, and major side effects of medications Verbalizes plans for follow-up care

Cardiac Arrhythmia

Nursing Diagnosis	Client Outcomes
Decreased cardiac output R/T effects of arrhythmia	Within ___: B/P WNL for client P strong, 60–100 beats/min Cardiac output ≥ ___
Pain R/T myocardial ischemia 2° rapid rate	Verbalizes decreased pain within ___ after administration of anti-ischemic/antiarrhythmic medication
Fear R/T potential life-threatening effects of arrhythmia, possibility of death	Verbalizes decreased fear within ___
Sleep pattern disturbance R/T critical care environment, recurrent rhythm disturbances	Sleeps at least ___ hours uninterrupted within ___
Fatigue R/T decreased cardiac output, recurrent rhythm disturbances	Verbalizes decreased fatigue within ___
Impaired physical mobility R/T fear of recurrent arrhythmia	Performs prearrhythmia activities with or without assistance prior to discharge
Altered thought processes R/T sensory overload, lack of sleep	When reoriented, correctly identifies person, place, and time
Knowledge deficit (arrhythmia, precipitating factors, medications, follow-up care)	Prior to discharge: Describes arrhythmia and identifies precipitating factors Names action, dosage, and major side effects of prescribed medications Explains importance of and states plans for follow-up care

Cardiac Catheterization

Nursing Diagnosis	Client Outcomes
Knowledge deficit (procedure, postprocedure care, medications)	Prior to procedure, states purpose of cardiac catheterization Prior to discharge: Demonstrates site care Correctly describes catheterization results and follow-up recommendations Names own medications and describes action, dosage, and major side effects Explains importance of and states plans for follow-up care
Decreased cardiac output R/T decreased myocardial perfusion, complications of procedure	Following procedure: B/P, heart rate/rhythm WNL for client No evidence of lethal dysrhythmias Alert, oriented q shift Urine output > 30 ml/hour
Altered cardiopulmonary, cerebral, and peripheral tissue perfusion R/T effects of clot formation, compromised circulation in extremity distal to catheter insertion	Following procedure: No evidence of coronary ischemia, respiratory distress Neurological signs WNL for client Strong, equal peripheral pulses Capillary refill time < 3 seconds Warm, dry extremities No evidence of bleeding, hematoma
Altered protection R/T effects of invasive procedure, contrast media	Following procedure: No evidence of complications associated with procedure

Text continued on following page

Cardiac Catheterization *Continued*

Nursing Diagnosis	Client Outcomes
Pain R/T prolonged bedrest, immobilized extremity, effects of procedure	Expresses comfort within ___ after initiation of comfort measures
Noncompliance with activity restrictions R/T lack of understanding of importance of bedrest and immobilization of extremity	Following procedure: Remains on bedrest for ___ hours with R/L extremity immobilized
Ineffective individual/family coping R/T misconceptions about procedure, probable outcome, potential for percutaneous transluminal coronary angioplasty (PTCA)/surgery	Prior to procedure, accurately describes procedure, risks Prior to discharge: Accurately describes outcome and planned interventions Identifies support systems and positive coping strategies
Situational low self-esteem R/T perceived loss of control, change in role, lack of support systems	Prior to discharge, verbalizes positive statements about self and abilities to manage necessary changes

Congestive Heart Failure

Nursing Diagnosis	Client Outcomes
Activity intolerance R/T dyspnea and fatigue	B/P, P, and R do not exceed recommended limits during activity
Fatigue R/T increased metabolic demands, hypoxia	Verbalizes decreased fatigue within ___
Decreased cardiac output R/T reduction in stroke volume	Within 24 hours after admission: B/P WNL for client, A/P 60–100/min No evidence of gallop rhythm R unlabored @ 16–22 minutes
High risk for aspiration R/T excessive secretions, effects of sedation	No evidence of aspiration throughout hospitalization
Impaired gas exchange R/T excessive pulmonary secretions, anxiety	Within 24 hours after admission: Respiratory rate, rhythm, and depth WNL for client ABG WNL for client Alert and oriented Clear breath sounds
Fluid volume excess R/T decreased cardiac output	Throughout hospitalization: B/P and P WNL for client No evidence of labored respirations or gallop rhythm Balanced I&O No evidence of jugular vein distention, edema Weight loss of at least ___ lb
Altered nutrition: less than body requirements R/T anorexia, nausea, fatigue	Weight loss no greater than ___ lb throughout hospitalization
High risk for impaired skin integrity R/T edema, decreased mobility, impaired tissue perfusion	Throughout hospitalization, no evidence of skin breakdown

Text continued on following page

Congestive Heart Failure *Continued*

Nursing Diagnosis	Client Outcomes
Altered oral mucous membrane R/T prolonged oxygen therapy	While receiving oxygen therapy, moist, intact oral mucous membrane
Bathing/hygiene self-care deficit R/T weakness, fatigue, dyspnea	Prior to discharge, bathes self with or without assistance
Constipation R/T decreased mobility, decreased food and/or fluid intake	Prior to discharge, resumes normal pattern of elimination q ___
Altered thought processes: confusion R/T decreased cerebral perfusion, sensory overload, lack of sleep	When reoriented, correctly identifies person, place, and time
High risk for trauma R/T syncope, dizziness, weakness	Throughout hospitalization, no evidence of accident or injury
Altered cerebral peripheral tissue perfusion R/T decreased cardiac output, edema	Within 48 hours: Edema less than 1 + Alert and oriented
Sleep pattern disturbance R/T nocturnal dyspnea, anxiety, hospital routine	Prior to discharge: Sleeps at least 4 uninterrupted hours q 24 hours Resumes usual sleep habits
Situational low self-esteem R/T increased dependence on others	Prior to discharge: Verbalizes positive abilities Identifies support systems
Inability to manage therapeutic regimen (individual) R/T lack of financial resources, complexity of therapeutic regimen, previous unsuccessful experience with advised regimen	Prior to discharge: Identifies available financial resources Explains the need for and identifies plans for implementing therapeutic regimen
Fear R/T probability of recurrence/death, dyspnea	Prior to discharge: Verbalizes decreased feelings of fear

Nursing Diagnosis	Client Outcomes
High risk for impaired home maintenance management R/T persistent fatigue	Prior to discharge, identifies alternative resources for home maintenance
Knowledge deficit (disease process, low-sodium diet, prescribed medications, cardiac risk factors)	Prior to discharge: Describes disease process Selects appropriate low-sodium foods from menu Verbalizes action, dosage, and major side effects of prescribed medications Lists personal risk factors and identifies strategies for reduction

Myocardial Infarction

Nursing Diagnosis	Client Outcomes
Activity intolerance R/T pain, fear of pain, fatigue	B/P, P, and R do not exceed recommended levels during activity
Colonic constipation R/T decreased mobility, decreased oral intake	Resumes normal bowel elimination pattern q __ before discharge
Decreased cardiac output R/T effects of ischemia	Within __ days: B/P WNL for client P strong, regular, 60–100 beats/min Cardiac output WNL for client
Pain R/T effects of ischemia	Expresses comfort within __ minutes after initiation of comfort measures
Ineffective breathing pattern R/T pain, effects of medications	Within __ No evidence of dyspnea Respiratory rate, depth, and rhythm WNL for client
Bathing self-care deficit R/T pain, dyspnea, fatigue	Prior to discharge, bathes self within physical limitations and activity restrictions
Altered sexuality patterns R/T pain, fear of recurrence, decreased self-esteem	Prior to discharge, verbalizes sexual adequacy and discusses potential alternative activities
Sleep pattern disturbance R/T anxiety, pain, hospital environment	Within __ days: Verbalizes feeling rested Sleeps minimum of 4 uninterrupted hours twice daily
Fear R/T possibility of death, severe pain, implications of diagnosis and treatment	Verbalizes feelings of decreased fearfulness within hours
Ineffective denial R/T perceived impact of disease process	Prior to discharge, acknowledges occurrence of myocardial infarction

Nursing Diagnosis	Client Outcomes
Ineffective individual (family) coping R/T perceived change in lifestyle	Prior to discharge, verbalizes positive approaches to deal with lifestyle changes
Altered family processes R/T perceived change in roles	Verbalizes methods of adapting to required role changes
Anticipatory grieving R/T perceived losses 2° cardiac dysfunction	Prior to discharge: Expresses feelings to person of choice Verbalizes diagnosis and actual limitations
Powerlessness R/T feelings of loss of control over life	Prior to discharge, verbalizes increased feelings of control
Situational low self-esteem R/T perceived changes in role	Prior to discharge, verbalizes positive statements about self and role changes
Knowledge deficit (disease process, risk factors, diet, activity, medications)	Prior to discharge: Describes the etiology of myocardial infarction Names own risk factors and identifies reduction strategies Selects low-sodium, low-fat, and low-cholesterol foods from menu Explains activity limitations and rate of progression Names action, dosage, and major side effects of prescribed medications

Pacemaker

Nursing Diagnosis	Client Outcomes
Preinsertion	
Decreased cardiac output R/T rhythm disturbance	Prior to insertion: Systolic B/P > 80 mmHg Palpable peripheral pulses
Fear R/T possible hazards associated with surgical procedure	Verbalizes decreased fear prior to surgery
Postinsertion	
Pain R/T effects of surgery, immobilization	Expresses comfort within minutes after initiation of comfort measure
High risk for infection R/T hazards associated with invasive procedure	No evidence of infection throughout hospitalization
Impaired physical mobility: L/R arm/shoulder R/T pain, anxiety	Full ROM of operative arm/ shoulder within 72 hours
Sleep pattern disturbance R/T anxiety, frequent monitoring, unfamiliar environment	Sleeps at least 4 uninterrupted hours twice daily Verbalizes feeling rested within ___ days
Ineffective individual coping R/T perceived lifestyle limitations	Prior to discharge, identifies positive coping strategies and available support systems
Impaired home maintenance management R/T fear of pacemaker malfunction	Prior to discharge, identifies alternative resources for home maintenance
Body image disturbance R/T change in cardiac function	Verbalizes positive statements about self prior to discharge
Knowledge deficit (pacemaker function, safety precautions, and follow-up care)	Prior to discharge: Verbalizes rationale for and function of pacemaker Takes own pulse Identifies safety precautions associated with pacemaker Verbalizes plan for follow-up care

Percutaneous Transluminal Coronary Angioplasty (PTCA)

Nursing Diagnosis	Client Outcomes
Pain R/T effects of ischemia, reocclusion, dysrhythmias	Reports pain promptly when experiencing it Verbalizes decreased pain within __ minutes after initiation of comfort measures
High risk for injury R/T hazards associated with procedure	Throughout hospitalization: No evidence of lethal dysrhythmia, reocclusion, tamponade, bleeding Vital signs, hemodynamic parameters WNL for client PTT 1–1.5 times control
Altered cerebral, peripheral tissue perfusion R/T hazards associated with procedure	Following procedure: Neurological signs WNL for client Strong, equal peripheral pulses Capillary refill time < 3 seconds Warm, dry skin
High risk for fluid volume deficit R/T decreased circulating blood volume 2° persistent bleeding, diuresis, high-volume contrast media	Within __ : B/P, hemodynamic parameters WNL for client Urine output > 125 ml/hour
Fear R/T threat of death, critical care environment, uncertain outcome, potential for reocclusion	Verbalizes decreased fear within __
High risk for infection R/T effects of invasive lines/procedures	No evidence of local/systemic infection throughout hospitalization
Ineffective denial R/T perceived resolution of coronary artery stenosis, lack of support systems	Prior to discharge, acknowledges presence of coronary artery disease

Text continued on following page

Percutaneous Transluminal Coronary Angioplasty (PTCA) *Continued*

Nursing Diagnosis	Client Outcomes
Ineffective management of therapeutic regimen R/T denial, perceived decrease in quality of life	Prior to discharge, verbalizes rationale for and states intention to follow recommended therapeutic regimen
Knowledge deficit (procedure, pre-/postprocedure care, follow-up care)	Prior to procedure, accurately describes procedure and pre-/postprocedure care Prior to discharge: Defines disease process Names own medications and describes action, dosage, and major side effects Identifies postdischarge resources Explains the importance of and states plans for follow-up care

D/D of the Digestive System

 Colostomy

Nursing Diagnosis	Client Outcomes
Preoperative	
Fear R/T uncertain diagnosis, outcome of surgery	Verbalizes decreased fear prior to surgery
Postoperative	
High risk for altered tissue integrity R/T decreased perfusion to stoma, contamination of wound by ostomy drainage/surgical drain	Following surgery: Dark pink or red stomal coloring Demonstrates wound healing prior to discharge
Pain R/T effects of surgery, N/G tube placement	Expresses comfort within 45 minutes after initiation of comfort measure
Altered sexuality patterns R/T negative self-concept, fear of rejection, possible accidental spillage	Prior to discharge, verbalizes sexual adequacy and expresses interest in adapting sexual patterns as necessary
High risk for impaired skin integrity R/T irritating stomal drainage	No evidence of redness, swelling, or excoriation at stomal site throughout hospitalization
Situational low self-esteem R/T change in body image	Prior to discharge, verbalizes positive feelings about self and plans to adapt to body image changes
Impaired social interaction R/T fear of rejection, accidental spillage, odor	Discusses plans to continue/resume participation in social activities prior to discharge
Altered individual (family) coping R/T change in body function, fear of rejection, inadequate support systems	Identifies positive strategies for coping with ostomy prior to discharge

Text continued on following page

Colostomy *Continued*

Nursing Diagnosis	Client Outcomes
Impaired adjustment R/T lack of financial resources, perceived stigma associated with ostomy	Verbalizes strategies and available support systems to assist in management of ostomy prior to discharge
High risk for injury R/T complications of surgical procedure, obstruction	No evidence of complications/obstruction throughout hospitalization
Knowledge deficit (care of ostomy, diet modifications, support systems, follow-up care)	By time of discharge, client/family: Demonstrates application of ostomy pouch Verbalizes diet modifications required to facilitate ostomy function Identifies available personal/community resources Explains the need for and describes plan for obtaining follow-up care

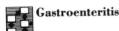 **Gastroenteritis**

Nursing Diagnosis	Client Outcomes
Fluid volume deficit R/T excessive fluid loss, decreased oral intake 2° vomiting/diarrhea, inability to absorb food/fluids	Within ___: Returns to hydration level WNL for client Balanced I&O
Diarrhea R/T effects of infectious process	Prior to discharge, resumes normal pattern of bowel elimination
Pain R/T abdominal cramping 2° increased gastrointestinal motility	Verbalizes comfort within ___ minutes after initiation of comfort measures
Fear R/T lack of knowledge of underlying disease process, diagnostic procedures	Verbalizes decreased fear within ___
High risk for altered nutrition: less than body requirements R/T nausea, vomiting, diarrhea	Weight loss no greater than ___ lb within ___
High risk for altered perianal skin integrity R/T contact with irritating liquid stools	No evidence of perianal skin breakdown throughout hospitalization
Altered oral mucous membranes R/T persistent vomiting, presence of N/G tube, decreased oral intake	Oral mucosa moist, pink, without ulceration throughout hospitalization
Bathing/toileting self-care deficit R/T weakness, fatigue	Bathes/toilets self with assistance by ___ Bathes/toilets self independently by ___
High risk for altered thought processes R/T effects of dehydration, electrolyte imbalance, unfamiliar environment	Remains oriented to person, place, and time throughout hospitalization

Text continued on following page

Gastroenteritis *Continued*

Nursing Diagnosis	Client Outcomes
Altered health maintenance R/T lack of knowledge of appropriate food/fluid intake, prevention of recurrence	Prior to discharge: Selects appropriate food/fluids from menu Identifies methods to prevent recurrence

Gastrointestinal Bleeding

Nursing Diagnosis	Client Outcomes
Fluid volume deficit R/T recurrent bleeding	Within ___ days: No evidence of dehydration, hypovolemia CVP WNL for client
High risk for altered peripheral tissue perfusion R/T decreased blood volume	Throughout hospitalization: Skin color WNL for client Normal capillary refill time
High risk for trauma R/T weakness, fatigue	Throughout hospitalization, no evidence of accident or injury
Altered nutrition: less than body requirements R/T NPO status, anorexia	Weight loss no greater than ___ lb throughout hospitalization
Altered oral mucous membrane R/T mouth breathing, N/G tube	Oral mucosa moist, pink, without ulceration while N/G tube in place
Impaired gas exchange R/T effects of decreased hemoglobin	Within ___ days: ABG WNL for client No evidence of hypoxia
High risk for aspiration R/T presence of gastrointestinal tubes, reduced level of consciousness, increased gastric residual	While gastrointestinal tubes in place: Lungs remain clear Afebrile Chest x-ray clear
Bathing/toileting self-care deficit R/T weakness, IV catheter placement	Bathes/toilets self with assistance, progressing to independence prior to discharge
High risk for impaired skin integrity R/T recurrent bloody liquid stools	No evidence of skin breakdown during hospitalization
Sleep pattern disturbance R/T effects of hospitalization, constant monitoring	Verbalizes feelings of restfulness within ___ days

Text continued on following page

Gastrointestinal Bleeding *Continued*

Nursing Diagnosis	Client Outcomes
Hypothermia R/T decreased blood volume, multiple transfusions of cold blood, iced saline irrigations	Temperature WNL within 48 hours
Altered patterns of urinary elimination R/T decreased oral intake, decreased renal perfusion	Voids at least 240 ml per shift
Fear R/T obvious bleeding, possibility of death outcome of surgery	Verbalizes decreased feelings of fearfulness within ___ hours
Altered thought processes: confusion R/T decreased cerebral flow, sensory overload	Alert and oriented to person, place, and time throughout hospitalization
Knowledge deficit (disease process, precipitating factors, diet, medications, follow-up care)	Prior to discharge: Explains disease process and precipitating factors Selects appropriate foods from menu Names actions, dosage, and major side effects of prescribed medications Explains the need for and describes plans for follow-up care

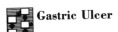 **Gastric Ulcer**

Nursing Diagnosis	Client Outcomes
Altered nutrition: less than body requirements R/T decreased oral intake, pain	Weight loss no greater than ___ lb during hospitalization
Pain R/T increased gastric secretions	Expresses comfort within ___ minutes after comfort measures
Activity intolerance R/T persistent fatigue, lack of sleep	Resumes normal ADL without fatigue prior to discharge
High risk for aspiration R/T side effects of N/G tube, increased gastric residual	Throughout hospitalization, no evidence of aspiration
High risk for trauma R/T weakness, fatigue, and pain	Throughout hospitalization, no evidence of accident or injury
Constipation R/T dietary changes, side effects of medications	Prior to discharge, resumes normal bowel elimination pattern q ___
Sleep pattern disturbance R/T nocturnal pain	Throughout hospitalization, experiences at least 4 hours of uninterrupted sleep twice q 24 hours
Fear R/T pain, diagnostic studies, unfamiliar environment	Verbalizes decreased feelings of fear within ___ hours
Ineffective denial R/T perceived impact of disease process	Prior to discharge: Acknowledges presence of ulcer disease
Knowledge deficit (disease process, diet, medication therapy, follow-up care)	Prior to discharge: Describes disease process Selects appropriate foods from menu States action, dosage, and major side effects of prescribed medications Identifies need for and describes planned follow-up care

D/D of the Hepatobiliary System

 Cholelithiasis/Cholecystitis

Nursing Diagnosis	Client Outcomes
Ineffective breathing pattern R/T effects of pain, fear, and anxiety	Respiratory rate, rhythm, and depth WNL for client within hours
Fluid volume deficit R/T vomiting, dehydration	Fluid intake of at least 3000 ml q 24 hours
Altered nutrition: less than body requirements R/T nausea, vomiting, anorexia	Throughout hospitalization, weight loss does not exceed ___ lb
Pain R/T inflammatory process, nausea, and vomiting	Expresses comfort within minutes after initiation of comfort measure
Altered oral mucous membrane R/T mouth breathing, dehydration	Throughout hospitalization: Moist mucous membranes No evidence of cracking or ulceration
Fear R/T recurrent pain, outcome of diagnostic studies	Verbalizes decreased fear within 24 hours
High risk for trauma R/T weakness, fatigue, postural hypotension	During hospitalization, no evidence of accident or injury
Knowledge deficit (disease process, diet, follow-up care)	Prior to discharge: Describes disease process Selects appropriate foods from menu Identifies the need for and describes plans for obtaining follow-up care

D/D of the Musculoskeletal System

 Back Pain

Nursing Diagnosis	Client Outcomes
Colonic constipation R/T decreased mobility, effects of medication	Resumes normal bowel elimination pattern q — prior to discharge
Chronic pain R/T effects of nerve impingement, recurrent muscle spasm	Expresses comfort within minutes after initiation of comfort measure
Impaired physical mobility R/T persistent pain, traction	During hospitalization, full ROM of nonaffected extremities
Altered sexuality patterns R/T fear of recurrent pain	Prior to discharge: Verbalizes concerns to person of choice Identifies alternative sexual approaches
High risk for impaired skin integrity R/T prolonged immobility	Throughout hospitalization, no evidence of skin breakdown over bony prominences
Sleep pattern disturbance R/T inability to assume usual position, pain	Experiences at least 4 hours of uninterrupted sleep twice q 24 hours
Altered patterns of urinary elimination R/T horizontal position, pain	Prior to discharge, resumes normal urinary elimination patterns
Fear R/T outcome of diagnostic procedures	Verbalizes decreased fear within 24 hours
Ineffective individual coping R/T limitations imposed by persistent pain	Prior to discharge, identifies positive coping strategies to deal with limitations
Impaired home maintenance management R/T recurrent back pain, physical limitations	Names alternatives for home maintenance prior to discharge

Text continued on following page

Back Pain *Continued*

Nursing Diagnosis	Client Outcomes
Knowledge deficit (disease process, activity limitations, lifestyle modifications)	Prior to discharge: Describes disease process Lists own activity limitations Identifies necessary lifestyle modifications

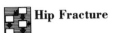 **Hip Fracture**

Nursing Diagnosis	Client Outcomes

Preoperative

Pain R/T inflammatory process, edema, effects of trauma	Expresses comfort within ___ minutes after initiation of comfort measure
Knowledge deficit (surgical experience, pre-/postoperative care)	Prior to surgery: Explains operative procedure Describes preoperative routine and anticipated postoperative care

Postoperative

Pain R/T inflammatory process, effects of surgery	Expresses comfort within ___ minutes after initiation of comfort measure
Impaired physical mobility R/T effects of pain, weakness, fear	Demonstrates sufficient muscle strength to cooperate with turning and ROM exercises in immediate postoperative period Prior to discharge, ambulates/transfers with or without assistance
High risk for disuse syndrome R/T effects of prolonged immobility	No evidence of body system deterioration/complications of immobility throughout hospitalization
Activity intolerance R/T prolonged immobility	B/P, P, R WNL for client in response to activity
High risk for infection R/T effects of anesthesia/surgical procedure, hazards associated with invasive equipment/procedures	No evidence of local/systemic infection throughout hospitalization
High risk for peripheral neurovascular dysfunction R/T effects of surgery	No evidence of peripheral neurovascular complications throughout hospitalization

Text continued on following page

Hip Fracture *Continued*

Nursing Diagnosis	Client Outcomes
Constipation R/T prolonged immobility, effects of aging	Resumes normal bowel pattern of q ___ prior to discharge
High risk for altered thought processes R/T effects of pain medication, unfamiliar environment, effects of decreased visual/hearing acuity	When reoriented, correctly identifies person, place, and time
Ineffective management of therapeutic regimen R/T lack of knowledge regarding postdischarge care	Prior to discharge, client/caregiver verbalizes discharge instructions regarding activity, care of incision, and medical therapy

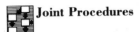 **Joint Procedures**

Nursing Diagnosis	Client Outcomes
Preoperative	
Pain R/T inflammatory process	Expresses comfort within 45 minutes after initiation of comfort measures
Knowledge deficit (surgical experience, postoperative care)	Prior to surgery: Explains operative procedure Describes preoperative routine and anticipated postoperative care
Postoperative	
Pain R/T effects of surgery, inflammatory process	Expresses comfort within 45 minutes after initiation of comfort measures
High risk for impaired skin integrity R/T prolonged immobility	No evidence of skin breakdown postoperatively
High risk for disuse syndrome R/T effects of prescribed immobility	No evidence of body system deterioration throughout hospitalization
Constipation R/T prolonged immobility	Resumes normal bowel patterns q __ before discharge
High risk for injury (dislocation) R/T effects of unstable joint	At time of discharge demonstrates healing with extremity in proper alignment
High risk for peripheral neurovascular dysfunctions R/T effects of surgery, immobilization	No evidence of peripheral neurovascular complications throughout hospitalization
High risk for infection R/T effects of anesthesia/ surgery, hazards associated with invasive equipment	Throughout hospitalization, no evidence of local/ systemic infection

Text continued on following page

Joint Procedures *Continued*

Nursing Diagnosis	Client Outcomes
Knowledge deficit (use of assistive devices, exercise, activity, rehabilitation, support systems, follow-up care)	Prior to discharge: Uses (specify) safely in ADL Demonstrates exercises and states daily frequency of each Explains activity limitations Describes recommended rehabilitation process Identifies available support systems Verbalizes need for and describes plans for follow-up care

D/D of the Skin, Subcutaneous Tissue, Breast

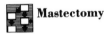 **Mastectomy**

Nursing Diagnosis	Client Outcomes
Pain R/T effects of surgery	Expresses comfort within __ minutes after comfort measure
Fluid volume excess R/T effects of surgery	No evidence of unusual edema in L/R arm throughout hospitalization
High risk for infection R/T effects of impaired vascular and lymphatic drainage	No evidence of wound infection throughout hospitalization
Impaired physical mobility: L/R arm R/T pain, lymphedema	Prior to discharge: Maximum ROM within limitations No evidence of unusual edema of arm
Altered sexuality patterns R/T fear of rejection by partner, perceived loss of femininity	Prior to discharge: Expresses concerns to person of choice Verbalizes sexual adequacy and plans to resume sexual activity
Fear R/T outcome of surgery, possibility of death, altered physical appearance	Verbalizes decreased fearfulness by time of discharge
Ineffective individual (family) coping R/T feelings about diagnosis of cancer, change in body image	Verbalizes feelings and identifies available support systems prior to discharge
Impaired adjustment R/T inability to accept changes in body image, perceived lack of support systems	Verbalizes positive approaches to assist in adjustment process prior to discharge
Anticipatory grieving R/T feelings about loss of breast	Prior to discharge: Verbalizes feelings about loss of breast

Text continued on following page

Mastectomy *Continued*

Nursing Diagnosis	Client Outcomes
Body image disturbance R/T changes in physical appearance	Prior to discharge: Expresses positive feelings about self
Impaired social interaction R/T fear of reactions/ rejection, own embarrassment	Prior to discharge: Verbalizes plan to resume social activities Identifies available support systems
Knowledge deficit (wound care, exercise, BSE, complications, support systems, follow-up care)	Prior to discharge: Demonstrates dressing change and wound care Performs hand, arm, and shoulder exercises as prescribed Verbalizes importance of BSE and performs examination in remaining breast Identifies potential complications and methods of prevention Lists available resources for prosthesis and support Verbalizes the need for and discusses plans for follow-up care

Endocrine, Nutritional, Metabolic Diseases

 Diabetes

Nursing Diagnosis	Client Outcomes
Fluid volume deficit R/T vomiting, diarrhea, decreased oral intake	Throughout hospitalization: No evidence of dehydration Balanced I & O No more than ___ stools q shift
Altered nutrition: less than body requirements R/T decreased oral intake, hypoglycemia	Weight loss no greater than ___ lb during hospitalization
High risk for impaired skin integrity R/T decreased mobility, increased blood sugar, decreased sensation	No evidence of skin breakdown during hospitalization
Reflex incontinence R/T loss of sphincter control 2° to neuropathy	Voids at least ___ ml q shift Decreased incidence of episodes of incontinence by time of discharge
High risk for infection R/T elevated blood glucose, decreased tissue perfusion	During hospitalization: Temperature, WBC WNL for client No evidence of infection
High risk for trauma R/T visual disturbances, neuropathy	No evidence of accident or injury during hospitalization
Sensory/perceptual alteration: tactile R/T effects of paresthesia, neuropathy	Verbalizes decreased burning, numbness, and tingling prior to discharge
Sensory perceptual alteration: visual R/T effects of disease process (retinopathy)	No evidence of progression of visual disturbances throughout hospitalization
Sexual dysfunction R/T peripheral neuropathy, altered self-concept	Prior to discharge, verbalizes beginning acceptance of changes in sexual patterns

Text continued on following page

Diabetes *Continued*

Nursing Diagnosis	Client Outcomes
Chronic low self-esteem R/T lifestyle changes, effects of chronic disease	Prior to discharge, expresses positive feelings about self and abilities
Anticipatory grieving R/T lifestyle changes, uncertain future	Prior to discharge, verbalizes feelings regarding lifestyle changes, prognosis
Ineffective management of therapeutic regimen (individual) R/T inability to incorporate necessary lifestyle changes	Prior to discharge, expresses intent to cooperate in treatment plan
Powerlessness R/T progressive nature of disease, complications	Prior to discharge, verbalizes increased feelings of control in managing disease process
Knowledge deficit (disease process, diet, exercise, medications, weight control, complications)	Prior to discharge: Describes disease process (diabetes) Selects appropriate foods for 1800-calorie ADA diet from menu Explains the role of exercise in treatment regimen Lists action, dosage, and major side effects of prescribed medications Identifies strategies for weight control Names the most common complications of diabetes and identifies methods of prevention

D/D of the Kidney and Urinary Tract

 Transurethral Resection of the Prostate (TURP)

Nursing Diagnosis	Client Outcomes
Preoperative	
Pain R/T effects of obstruction secondary to enlarged prostate	Verbalizes comfort within ___ minutes after initiation of comfort measure
Knowledge deficit (surgical experience, pre-/postoperative care)	Prior to surgery: Explains operative procedure Describes preoperative routine and anticipated postoperative care
Fear R/T unknown outcome of surgery, possible sexual dysfunction	Verbalizes decreased fear prior to surgery
Postoperative	
Pain (bladder spasm) R/T effects of surgical procedure, bladder irrigation, presence of clots	Expresses comfort within ___ minutes after initiation of comfort measure
High risk for injury (hemorrhage) R/T effects of surgery	No evidence of hemorrhage throughout postoperative period
High risk for infection R/T effects of invasive procedure, indwelling catheter	No evidence of infection throughout hospitalization
Altered patterns of urinary elimination R/T effects of impaired sphincter control secondary to surgery	Prior to discharge, reports decreased or absent urinary dribbling
Knowledge deficit (postoperative complications, activity restrictions, follow-up care)	Prior to discharge: Identifies postoperative complications and describes methods of prevention Explains activity limitations Describes the importance of and states plans for follow-up care

Acute Urinary Tract Infection

Nursing Diagnosis	Client Outcomes
Hyperthermia R/T effects of infectious process	Temperature WNL for client within ___
Pain R/T dysuria, effects of bladder spasms, inflammatory process	Verbalizes comfort within ___ minutes after initiation of comfort measures
Altered patterns of urinary elimination R/T effects of infectious process	Prior to discharge: Verbalizes decreased/absent symptoms Return to preinfection pattern of urinary elimination
Knowledge deficit (disease process, risk of recurrent infection, preventive measures, medications, importance of adhering to therapeutic regimen)	Prior to discharge: Describes disease process Explains the risk of recurrent infection and describes the role of hygiene and urination habits in prevention Lists action, dosage, and major side effects of medications Discusses the importance of forcing fluids Describes the importance of adhering to the therapeutic regimen and identifies plans for follow-up care

Pregnancy, Childbirth, and Puerperium

 Cesarean Birth

Nursing Diagnosis	Client Outcomes
Constipation R/T effects of surgery/medications decreased mobility	Bowel movement by __ postoperative day
Pain R/T effects of surgery, breast engorgement, uterine contraction	Expresses comfort within __ minutes after initiation of comfort measure
High risk for fluid volume deficit R/T decreased oral intake, excessive vaginal bleeding	Intake of at least __ ml of fluid within 24 hours Vital signs WNL Vaginal bleeding less than __ pads/shift
High risk for infection R/T effects of surgery, breast engorgement, breast feeding	Throughout hospitalization: Temperature WNL No evidence of infection
High risk for altered nutrition: less than body requirements R/T decreased oral intake, increased metabolic demands 2° surgery, breastfeeding	Consumes at least __ calories daily Selects appropriate foods from menu prior to discharge
Altered sexuality patterns R/T fear of pregnancy, pain	Prior to discharge, verbalizes plan to resume normal sexual pattern within __ weeks postpartum
Sleep pattern disturbance R/T hospital routines, demands of newborn, pain, anxiety	Experiences at least __ hours of uninterrupted sleep each night Verbalizes decreased fatigue within __ days
Urinary retention R/T effects of surgery	Voids 180–200 ml at one time within 6–12 hours after delivery

Text continued on following page

Cesarean Birth *Continued*

Nursing Diagnosis	Client Outcomes
Effective breastfeeding R/T previous positive experience, maternal confidence, family/other support systems	Verbalizes satisfaction with breastfeeding process Infant weight gain of ___ lb/month
Ineffective breastfeeding R/T lack of knowledge about effective technique	Describes and demonstrates correct breastfeeding techniques within ___
Interrupted breastfeeding R/T maternal illness	Resumes breastfeeding pattern prior to discharge or Verbalizes feelings about discontinuing breastfeeding
Altered family processes R/T arrival of new member	Prior to discharge: Discusses changing roles of family members Describes plan for assimilation of new member
Altered parenting R/T separation from infant, inexperience, lack of role model	Prior to discharge: Verbalizes positive statements about abilities to care for infant Attends parenting class
Body image disturbance R/T changes associated with pregnancy, cesarean birth	Prior to discharge: Verbalizes positive feelings about self Lists strategies to ensure weight loss and increased muscle tone
Knowledge deficit (incisional care, newborn care, birth control)	Prior to discharge: Demonstrates wound care Demonstrates newborn care/feeding, bathing, diapering Identifies birth control method of choice

Normal Vaginal Delivery: Postpartum

Nursing Diagnosis	Client Outcomes
Pain R/T edema 2° to episiotomy, uterine contractions, breast engorgement	Expresses comfort within ___ minutes after initiation of comfort measure
High risk for infection R/T trauma associated with delivery, episiotomy	Throughout hospitalization: Temperature WNL No evidence of infection
Urinary retention R/T edema, pain, trauma associated with delivery	Voids 180–200 ml at one time within 6–12 hours after delivery
Constipation R/T pain, fear of pain, decreased oral intake, decreased mobility	Bowel movement by ___ postpartum day
High risk for fluid volume deficit R/T excessive vaginal bleeding	Throughout hospitalization: Vital signs WNL Vaginal bleeding less than ___ pads/shift
High risk for sleep pattern disturbance R/T demands of newborn, hospital routine	During hospitalization: Verbalizes decreased fatigue Sleeps at least 3 uninterrupted hours three times daily
Effective breastfeeding R/T previous positive experience, maternal confidence, family/other support systems	Verbalizes satisfaction with breastfeeding process Infant weight gain of ___ lb/month
Ineffective breastfeeding R/T separation from infant, nonsupportive spouse	Verbalizes plan for continued breastfeeding prior to discharge
High risk for interrupted breastfeeding R/T demand of maternal employment	Verbalizes strategies to facilitate continuation of breastfeeding prior to discharge
High risk for altered parenting R/T lack of parent-infant attachment	Prior to discharge: Verbalizes positively about infant Calls infant by name, touches and establishes eye contact

Text continued on following page

Normal Vaginal Delivery: Postpartum *Continued*

Nursing Diagnosis	Client Outcomes
Fear R/T parental role assumption	Verbalizes decreased fear prior to discharge
Altered family processes R/T arrival of new member	Prior to discharge, discusses changing roles of family members and describes plans for assimilation of new member
Body image disturbance R/T changes associated with pregnancy	Prior to discharge: Verbalizes positive feeling about self Lists strategies to ensure weight loss and muscle tone
Altered sexuality patterns R/T fear of pregnancy, pain	Prior to discharge, verbalizes plans to resume usual sexual patterns within ___ weeks postpartum
Knowledge deficit (newborn care)	Prior to discharge, demonstrates newborn care (e.g., bathing, diapering, feeding)

Newborns and Other Neonates with Conditions Originating in the Perinatal Period

 High-Risk Newborn (Prematurity, Large for Gestational Age, Small for Gestational Age)

Nursing Diagnosis	Client Outcomes
Activity intolerance R/T fatigue, dyspnea, trauma associated with delivery	B/P, P WNL during periods of activity
Ineffective airway clearance R/T diminished cough, excessive or retained secretions	No evidence of respiratory distress or obstruction q shift
Constipation R/T decreased fluid intake, bowel motility, mobility	Bowel movement within ___ days
Diarrhea R/T exposure to bacteria, effects of medication	No more than ___ stools per shift
Fluid volume deficit R/T decreased fluid intake, diarrhea	Intake of at least ___ ml of fluid q 8 hours
Ineffective breathing pattern R/T complicated delivery, effects of anesthesia, immaturity	Respiratory rate, rhythm, and depth WNL q shift
Impaired gas exchange R/T effects of immature alveoli, meconium or other aspiration, congenital abnormality	ABG WNL q ___
High risk for infection R/T effects of lack of normal flora, protective vernix	No evidence of infection throughout hospitalization
Altered nutrition: less than body requirements R/T decreased sucking, impaired swallowing, immaturity	Weight loss less than ___ oz q ___ Consumes at least ___ calories per shift

Text continued on following page

High-Risk Newborn (Prematurity, Large for Gestational Age, Small for Gestational Age)
Continued

Nursing Diagnosis	Client Outcomes
Ineffective infant feeding pattern R/T effects of immaturity, decreased infant sucking reflex	Weight gain of __ oz within __ days
High risk for altered skin integrity R/T lack of skin flora, protective vernix	No evidence of skin breakdown throughout hospitalization
High risk for aspiration R/T immaturity, effects of congenital defects	No evidence of aspiration throughout hospitalization
Ineffective thermoregulation R/T effects of immaturity	Body temperature between __ and __ degrees q shift
Altered family processes R/T effects of prolonged hospitalization on family	Family members verbalize feelings to person of choice before discharge
Anticipatory grieving: parental R/T potential loss, defects, or chronic illness of infant	Prior to discharge, family members: Express feelings regarding potential outcome(s) Identify positive coping strategies Identify available support systems
Altered growth and development R/T effects of immaturity, chronic disease, sensorimotor deficits	Age-appropriate growth and development
Altered parenting R/T impaired infant-parent attachment, feeling of maternal guilt, anxiety	Within __ hours: Parents express feelings about infant, potential outcome, role Parents call infant by name, touch infant, participate in care

Nursing Diagnosis	Client Outcomes
High risk for trauma, suffocation, poisoning R/T effects of immaturity, dependence on caregiver, environmental hazards	No evidence of accident or injury throughout hospitalization
Knowledge deficit (newborn care)	Prior to discharge, mother demonstrates newborn care (e.g., bathing, diapering, feeding)
High risk for caregiver role strain R/T inexperience, lack of confidence in abilities	Prior to discharge, caregiver: Verbalizes strategies to manage infant care Identifies family/community support systems

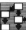 **Normal Newborn**

Nursing Diagnosis	Client Outcomes
High risk for aspiration R/T copious secretions	No evidence of aspiration throughout hospitalization
Hypothermia R/T exposure to cool environment	Temperature WNL q shift
Constipation R/T decreased fluid intake, formula	Bowel movement within ___
Diarrhea R/T exposure to bacteria, breast feeding	No more than ___ stools daily
Ineffective breathing pattern R/T effects of delivery, anesthesia, aspiration	Respiratory rate, rhythm, and depth WNL q shift
Fluid volume deficit R/T decreased oral intake, diarrhea	Intake of at least ___ ml q shift
High risk for infection R/T lack of normal flora, exposure to environmental hazards	No evidence of infection during postnatal period
Altered nutrition: less than body requirements R/T decreased sucking ability, formula intolerance, decreased availability of breast milk	Weight loss less than ___ oz per ___
Effective breastfeeding R/T previous positive experience, maternal confidence, family/other support systems	Verbalizes satisfaction with breastfeeding process Infant weight gain of ___ lb/month
Ineffective breastfeeding R/T maternal anxiety, weak infant sucking	Mother demonstrates effective breastfeeding techniques following instruction
High risk for altered growth and development R/T lack of parent-infant attachment, environmental stimulation	Age-appropriate growth and development

Nursing Diagnosis	Client Outcomes
High risk for trauma, suffocation, poisoning R/T lack of supervision by caregiver, environmental hazards	No evidence of accident, injury during postnatal period

Myeloproliferative D/D, Poorly Differentiated Neoplasms

 Terminal Cancer

Nursing Diagnosis	Client Outcomes
Ineffective breathing pattern R/T fear, pain, effects of analgesics	Rate, rhythm, and depth of R normal for client throughout hospitalization
High risk for aspiration R/T weak cough, viscous secretions	No evidence of aspiration throughout hospitalization
Fluid volume deficit R/T decreased oral intake, increased fluid loss	Within ___ hours, normal skin turgor, stable B/P, P, balanced I&O
Chronic pain R/T effects of disease process, medical regimen	Expresses comfort within ___ minutes after initiation of comfort measure
Impaired skin integrity R/T prolonged immobility	No evidence of skin breakdown throughout hospitalization
Altered protection R/T decreased nutritional status, altered blood profiles, hazards/effects of drug therapy, treatments, disease process	No evidence of hazards associated with decreased protective mechanisms (specify)
Altered oral mucous membrane R/T effects of chemotherapy	Moist, pink mucous membrane without cracking or ulceration throughout hospitalization
Impaired physical mobility R/T fatigue, weakness, dyspnea, motor deficits	During hospitalization, achieves maximum mobility within limitations of terminal state
Self-care deficit (specify) R/T progressive physical debilitation, weakness	During hospitalization, performs self-care activities within physical limitations

Nursing Diagnosis	Client Outcomes
Constipation R/T decreased mobility, fluid intake, obstructive process	During terminal phase of illness, achieves bowel routine that provides optimal comfort
Bowel incontinence R/T decreased level of consciousness, neurological deficit 2° disease process	Experiences absence or decreased episodes of incontinence q 24 hours
High risk for disuse syndrome R/T pain, immobility	No evidence of body system deterioration during hospitalization
Sleep pattern disturbance R/T anxiety, chronic pain, orthopnea	Experiences at least ___ hours of uninterrupted sleep/rest q 24 hours
Altered nutrition: less than body requirements R/T anorexia, nausea, and vomiting	Consumes at least ___ calories q 24 hours
Fear R/T imminent death, loss of loved ones, loss of control	During hospitalization, client/family verbalizes decreasing fear
Altered thought processes (confusion) R/T effects of medications, fluid/electrolyte imbalance	When oriented, identifies correct time, place, person
Ineffective individual/family coping R/T excessive anxiety, anticipatory grief, lack of support systems	Prior to death, client/family: Verbalizes effective coping strategies Identifies support systems
Impaired family adjustment R/T perceived outcome of illness, prolonged hospitalization	Prior to client's death, family verbalizes positive strategies to facilitate adjustment
Powerlessness R/T perceived inability to control progression of disease	Verbalizes increasing feelings of control of own response to disease process before death

Text continued on following page

Terminal Cancer *Continued*

Nursing Diagnosis	Client Outcomes
Spiritual distress R/T inability to practice spiritual rituals	Within ___ days, verbalizes alternative methods of completing spiritual practices
High risk for trauma R/T increasing weakness, altered thought processes	Throughout hospitalization, no evidence of accident or injury
High risk for infection R/T decreased immune response, presence of indwelling catheters/ invasive lines	Prior to death, no evidence of infection
Caregiver role strain R/T effects of prolonged/critical illness	Caregiver verbalizes strategies to deal with stresses associated with role
Knowledge deficit (disease process, outcome of illness, support systems, pain regimen)	Prior to client's death: Describes disease process Discusses prognosis Identifies available personal/ community support systems Describes action, dosage, and major side effects of prescribed pain medications

Infectious and Parasitic Diseases

 Acquired Immune Deficiency Syndrome (AIDS)

Nursing Diagnosis	Client Outcomes
Chronic pain R/T inflammatory process	Expresses comfort within 45 minutes after initiation of comfort measures
High risk for altered oral mucous membrane R/T secondary infection	No evidence of inflammation, ulceration throughout hospitalization
Altered nutrition: less than body requirements R/T anorexia, N/V, dehydration, effects of medication	Weight loss not greater than ___ lb within ___
Ineffective airway clearance R/T retained secretions, fatigue	No evidence of respiratory distress during hospitalization
Altered protection R/T decreased nutritional status, altered blood profiles, hazards/effects of drug therapy, treatments, disease process	No evidence of hazards associated with decreased protective mechanisms (specify)
High risk for disuse syndrome R/T disease process, effects of prolonged immobility	No evidence of deterioration of body systems throughout hospitalization
Impaired skin integrity R/T decreased mobility, altered nutritional status, incontinence	During hospitalization, no evidence of skin breakdown over bony prominences
Hyperthermia R/T infectious process, effects of medications	Temperature WNL within ___ hours
High risk for trauma R/T weakness, fatigue	No evidence of accident or injury during hospitalization

Text continued on following page

Acquired Immune Deficiency Syndrome (AIDS)
Continued

Nursing Diagnosis	Client Outcomes
Activity intolerance R/T fatigue, prolonged immobility, effects of debilitating disease	B/P and P WNL for client during periods of activity
Fatigue R/T increased energy requirements/decreased metabolic energy production	Verbalizes decreased fatigue within __
Fluid volume deficit R/T decreased oral intake, anorexia	Throughout hospitalization: No evidence of dehydration B/P and P WNL for client
High risk for infection R/T decreased immune response	No evidence of secondary/ opportunistic infection throughout hospitalization
Fear R/T imminent death, loss of loved ones, loss of control	Verbalizes decreased fear within __ hours
Ineffective individual (family) coping R/T stigma associated with disease	Identifies positive strategies for dealing with effects of diagnosis prior to discharge
Ineffective denial R/T effects of catastrophic incurable illness	Before discharge, names disease and discusses prognosis
Sensory/perceptual alterations (visual) R/T effects of disease process, medications	No evidence of progression of visual disturbance throughout hospitalization
Powerlessness R/T inability to control progress of disease	Verbalizes increased feelings of control over remaining lifetime before discharge
Social isolation R/T fear of transmission to others, stigma associated with disease	Verbalizes decreased loneliness and feelings of isolation before discharge

Nursing Diagnosis	Client Outcomes
Body image disturbance R/T feelings about wasting, disfiguring lesions	Verbalizes feelings about body changes to person of choice before discharge
Chronic low self-esteem R/T effects of chronic disease	Verbalizes positive statements about self and/or achievements before death
Altered thought processes (confusion) R/T effects of infectious complications 2° disease process	When reoriented, identifies correct person, place, time
High risk for caregiver role strain R/T inexperience of caregiver, lack of support systems	Prior to discharge, caregiver: Demonstrates skills required for client care Identifies support systems
Ineffective management of therapeutic regimen (individual) R/T complexity of treatment plan	Prior to discharge, client/ caregiver: Correctly describes components of treatment plan Demonstrates skills required to implement plan
Knowledge deficit (disease process, transmission, opportunistic infections, support systems, follow-up care)	Prior to discharge: Describes disease process and methods of transmission Identifies methods to decrease risk of opportunistic infections Names available support systems Explains the need for and describes plans for follow-up care

Septicemia

Nursing Diagnosis	Client Outcomes
High risk for altered cerebral, gastrointestinal, cerebral tissue perfusion R/T infectious process	Throughout hospitalization: No evidence of deteriorating neurological signs Bowel sounds, abdominal girth WNL for client Free of chest pain, dysrhythmias
Decreased cardiac output R/T effects of infectious process	Within ___ days: B/P WNL for client Pulse strong, regular, 60–100 beats/min Cardiac output ≥ ___
Altered thought processes R/T decreased cerebral perfusion	Maintains prehospitalization level of orientation
Altered protection R/T decreased immune response, hospital environment, effects of invasive procedure, medication therapy	No evidence of complications, secondary infection throughout hospitalization
Hyperthermia R/T effects of infectious process	Temperature WNL for client within ___ days
Fluid volume deficit R/T decreased oral intake, persistent hyperthermia	Within ___ days: No evidence of dehydration, hypovolemia B/P, P WNL for client
Fear R/T effects of hospital environment, perceived negative outcome, potential complications of therapy	Within ___ verbalizes decreased fear
Knowledge deficit (disease process, transmission, treatment regimen, follow-up care)	Prior to discharge: Describes disease process and method of transmission Explains recommended treatment regimen Identifies the need for and describes plans for follow-up care

Mental D/D

 Alzheimer's Disease

Nursing Diagnosis	Client Outcomes
Bowel incontinence R/T decreased awareness of urge to defecate, confusion, immobility	Within ___ no episodes of incontinence
Diversional activity deficit R/T inability to concentrate/perform visual activities	Participates in previous/new activities at least ___ times per ___
High risk for trauma R/T decreased perception of environment, unsteady gait, impaired judgment	No evidence of accident or injury throughout hospitalization
Impaired physical mobility R/T effects of debilitating disease	Full ROM in all extremities before discharge
Altered nutrition: less than body requirements R/T confusion, memory lapses, anorexia, decreased oral intake	Weight loss less than ___ lb q week
Dressing/grooming self-care deficit R/T confusion, effects of disease	Dresses and grooms independently or with assistance while able Identifies alternative caretaker prior to discharge
Sleep pattern disturbance R/T unfamiliar environment, confusion, overstimulation	Experiences at least ___ hours of uninterrupted sleep q 24 hours
Altered thought processes R/T confusion, decreased problem-solving abilities, anxiety	When reoriented, identifies correct person, place, time
Impaired adjustment R/T inability to accept effects of chronic disease	Within ___ after diagnosis: Verbalizes feelings about disease

Text continued on following page

Alzheimer's Disease *Continued*

Nursing Diagnosis	Client Outcomes
	Identifies positive strategies to adjust to disease
Anxiety R/T outcome of disease, perceived threat to self-concept	Verbalizes decreased anxiety within ___ days
Impaired verbal communication R/T confusion, memory deficit, preoccupation with disease	Communicates needs effectively when oriented
Ineffective family coping: compromised R/T effects of dealing with ill family member	Prior to discharge, family members: Verbalize feelings regarding ill family member Identify positive strategies to deal with effects of disease
Altered family processes R/T change in roles 2° chronic illness	Prior to discharge, family members: Identify changes in role precipitated by illness Verbalize feelings about change Identify methods of dealing with changes
Hopelessness R/T perceived inability to control progression of disease	Expresses positive feelings regarding those facets of lifestyle within control before discharge
Powerlessness R/T perceived loss of control over symptoms, lifestyle	Prior to discharge: Verbalizes feelings regarding loss of control Identifies abilities to control other components of lifestyle
Impaired social interaction R/T inability to communicate effectively, embarrassment, decreased mobility	Interacts with others at least ___ times per ___

Nursing Diagnosis	Client Outcomes
Ineffective management of therapeutic regimen (individual) R/T changes in sensorium, lack of support systems, need for caretaker	Follows recommended treatment regimen while able Identifies support systems, alternative caretaker when necessary
High risk for caregiver role strain R/T illness of caregiver, lack of respite for caregiver	Prior to discharge, caregiver: Identifies strategies to manage continued care of client
Relocation stress syndrome R/T lack of preparation for move, confusion	Within ___ days after transfer: Verbalizes decreased stress in new environment
Knowledge deficit (disease process, treatment, medications, available resources)	Prior to discharge, client/ family/caretaker: Describes disease process Explains recommended treatment regimen Names action, dosage, and major side effects of prescribed medications Identifies available personal, financial, and community resources

Depression

Nursing Diagnosis	Client Outcomes
Colonic constipation R/T anorexia, decreased oral intake, decreased activity, medication	Prior to discharge: resumes normal elimination patterns q __
Altered nutrition: less than body requirements R/T anorexia, lack of interest, preoccupation with illness	During hospitalization, no evidence of weight loss greater than __ lb
Altered nutrition: more than body requirements R/T imbalance between excessive intake and low activity/exercise	Prior to discharge, weight loss of at least __ lb
Dressing/grooming self-care deficit R/T feelings of worthlessness, decreased self-esteem, preoccupation with illness, low energy level	Dresses and grooms with or without assistance before discharge
Fatigue R/T preoccupation with self/psychological demands	Participates in ADL without reports of fatigue
Sexual dysfunction R/T decreased self-esteem, loss of interest, fear of rejection, effects of sexual abuse	Verbalizes positive statements regarding sexual abilities before discharge
Sleep pattern disturbance R/T hospitalization, early awakening, constant arousal	Within 72 hours, experiences at least 4 hours of uninterrupted sleep twice daily
Impaired adjustment R/T inability to accept loss of loved one, effects of chronic disease/trauma	Prior to discharge: Verbalizes feelings regarding (specify) Identifies strategies to facilitate adjustment to loss, disease, trauma

Nursing Diagnosis	Client Outcomes
Anxiety R/T perceived threat to personal safety, self-concept	Verbalizes decreased feelings of anxiety within __ days
Ineffective management of therapeutic regimen (individual) R/T denial of illness, lack of financial resources, lack of supervision	Prior to discharge: Verbalizes intent to implement medical regimen Identifies personal/financial resources
Post-trauma response R/T effects of war experience, fire, flood, MVA	Prior to discharge: Associates feelings with traumatic event Expresses feelings to person of choice Identifies resources for follow-up care
Ineffective individual coping R/T feelings of guilt, perceived rejection by family or coworkers, inability to express feelings, ineffective role modeling	Prior to discharge, identifies positive strategies to cope with identified stressors
Altered family processes R/T hospitalization, change in roles of members	Prior to discharge, family verbalizes changing role of members
Fear R/T concerns for own safety secondary to treatment regimen, other clients, loss of control	Verbalizes decreased feelings of fear within __ days
Dysfunctional grieving R/T inability to accept loss of significant other, body part/function, terminal/chronic illness	Prior to discharge: Verbalizes feeling regarding loss, illness to person of choice Identifies positive coping strategies
Hopelessness R/T feelings of worthlessness, perceived loss of control	Prior to discharge, verbalizes positive feelings about self and control of lifestyle
Powerlessness R/T low self-esteem, perceived lack of support systems/control	Prior to discharge, verbalizes ability to control own life, make decisions

Text continued on following page

Depression *Continued*

Nursing Diagnosis	Client Outcomes
Chronic low self-esteem R/T feelings of guilt, worthlessness, history of abuse, trauma	Prior to discharge, verbalizes positive feelings about self and abilities to achieve future goals
Impaired social interaction R/T feelings of worthlessness, fear of rejection	Prior to discharge, spends at least ___ minutes per day interacting with others
Social isolation R/T low energy levels, desire to withdraw from others	Prior to discharge: Participates in unit activities Spends at least ___ minutes out of room q shift
Altered thought processes R/T memory loss, inability to concentrate, decreased comprehension and response	Prior to discharge: Oriented to person, place, and time Concentrates on one project for at least ___ minutes Responds immediately and appropriately to questions
High risk for self-mutilation R/T feelings of hopelessness, helplessness, loneliness, anger	No incidents of self-mutilation during hospitalization
Diversional activity deficit R/T lack of interest in previously rewarding activities, limited environmental stimulation	Prior to discharge, demonstrates interest in activity of preference
High risk for injury R/T inability to concentrate, decreased attention to environment, suicidal ideation, command hallucinations	No evidence of accident or injury throughout hospitalization

Nursing Diagnosis	Client Outcomes
Knowledge deficit (disease process, treatment options, medications, support systems, follow-up care)	Prior to discharge: Describes depression etiology and contributing factors Identifies potential treatment options Describes action, dosage, and major side effects of medications Identifies personal, financial, and community support systems Explains the importance of and identifies plans for follow-up care

Psychoses

Nursing Diagnosis	Client Outcomes
Colonic constipation R/T effects of medication, decreased oral intake, immobility, retention of bowel contents	Bowel movement within ___ Resumes normal pattern of elimination within ___
Impaired physical mobility R/T effects of medication, weakness, withdrawal, need for restraints	Throughout hospitalization: Full ROM of all extremities Increases ambulation/activity as condition permits
Altered nutrition: less than body requirements R/T fear of poisoning, anorexia, hoarding	Weight loss less than ___ lb per ___ (time frame)
Altered nutrition: more than body requirements R/T imbalance between excessive food intake and decreased activity/exercise, effects of tranquilizers	Weight loss of at least ___ lb per ___ (time frame)
Bathing/hygiene self-care deficit R/T inability to recognize personal needs, prolonged dependence on others for direction	Bathes self with or without assistance during hospitalization
Sexual dysfunction R/T decreased self-esteem, lack of interest, effects of medication, fear of rejection	Prior to discharge: Verbalizes positive feelings regarding sexual ability, appeal Identifies plan to resume normal sexual activities
Sleep pattern disturbance R/T auditory/visual hallucinations, hyperactivity	Experiences at least ___ hours of uninterrupted sleep q 24 hours
Impaired adjustment R/T inability to recognize inappropriate behavior, feelings of hopelessness, helplessness	Prior to discharge: Verbalizes feelings regarding diagnosis and symptoms Identifies strategies to facilitate adjustment to disease, symptoms

Nursing Diagnosis	Client Outcomes
Defensive coping R/T impaired perception of reality, self-destructive behaviors	Prior to discharge: Verbalizes feelings to person of choice Identifies positive strategies to manage own defensive behavior
Ineffective family coping: disabling R/T effects of acute/chronic illness in family member, stigma of mental illness	Prior to discharge, family members: Express feelings about illness and stigma Identify positive strategies to deal with effects of illness of family member
Altered family processes R/T effects of long-term hospitalization of family member, depletion of financial resources, stigma of illness, uncertainty of outcome	Prior to discharge, family members: Describe effects of illness on family roles, routines List methods of dealing with effects of illness
Anxiety R/T inability to distinguish between reality and hallucinations/ delusions, recurrence of psychotic episode	Expresses decreased anxiety within ___
Hopelessness R/T perceived loss of control, potential for recurrence, effects of chronic disease	Prior to discharge, verbalizes positive feelings regarding self and abilities to manage lifestyle with or without assistance
Ineffective management of therapeutic regimen (individual) R/T impaired perception of reality, denial of need for medication, lack of financial resources, lack of supervision	Prior to discharge: Verbalizes plans to implement recommended treatment plan Lists available support systems
Powerlessness R/T effects of hospitalization/institu-tionalization, lack of support systems, effects of chronic mental illness	During hospitalization, identifies feelings of control over lifestyle

Text continued on following page

Psychoses *Continued*

Nursing Diagnosis	Client Outcomes
Self-esteem disturbance R/T feelings of alienation, inadequacy, stigma of mental illness	Prior to discharge, identifies positive feelings about self and abilities
Sensory/perceptual alterations (specify) R/T hallucinations, delusions, impaired perception of reality	Prior to discharge: No evidence of hallucinations, delusions Oriented to time, place, person
Impaired social interaction R/T inattention, impaired perception of reality, fear of rejection	Participates in at least ___ interactions with others each ___ (time frame)
Social isolation R/T mistrust, suspicion, preoccupation with hallucinations/delusions	Prior to discharge: Participates in unit activities Spends at least ___ minutes out of room q shift
High risk for violence: self-directed or directed toward others R/T inability to identify reality	Initiates no attempts to injure self or others each day
Diversional activity deficit R/T preoccupation with hallucinations, inability to concentrate	Resumes participation in previous/new activities within ___
Impaired home maintenance management R/T inability to make decisions, dependency on others, lack of financial resources	Prior to discharge identifies a plan to maintain living environment
High risk for injury R/T command hallucinations, effects of medications, destructive/violent behavior, suicidal ideation	No evidence of accident or injury during hospitalization

Nursing Diagnosis	Client Outcomes
Knowledge deficit (effects of medications, community support systems, drug/alcohol/food interactions, stress management techniques, follow-up care)	Prior to discharge: Describes action, dosage, and major side effects of medications Identifies community support systems Identifies stress-management techniques Lists drug/alcohol/food interactions to avoid Explains the importance of and identifies plans for follow-up care

Substance Abuse and Substance-Induced Organic Mental Disorders

 Substance Abuse

Nursing Diagnosis	Client Outcomes
Pain R/T effects of withdrawal process	Expresses comfort within 30 minutes after initiation of comfort measure
Fluid volume deficit R/T decreased oral intake, vomiting, diarrhea	Consumes at least ___ ml of fluid each 24 hours
Constipation R/T decreased oral intake, lack of exercise, side effects of drugs	Resumes normal bowel pattern q ___ within ___ days
Diarrhea R/T effects of withdrawal process, anxiety	Resumes normal bowel pattern q ___ within ___ days
Altered nutrition: less than body requirements R/T anorexia, lack of concern about nutritional intake	Weight loss less than ___ lb per ___ (time frame)
Dressing/grooming self-care deficit R/T effects of withdrawal or intoxication	Dresses/grooms with or without assistance daily
Sleep pattern disturbance R/T effects of intoxication, withdrawal, sleep deprivation, irritability, anxiety	Experiences at least 4 hours of uninterrupted sleep q 24 hours
High risk for altered skin integrity R/T repeated self-injection, dehydration	No evidence of skin breakdown throughout hospitalization
Impaired adjustment R/T lack of confidence in abilities to remain substance-free, denial of addiction	Prior to discharge: Verbalizes feelings regarding (specify) Identifies strategies to facilitate adjustment

Nursing Diagnosis	Client Outcomes
Anxiety R/T perceived loss of control, effects of hospitalization, withdrawal process, absence of drugs/alcohol	Verbalizes decreased feelings of anxiety within __ days
Ineffective individual coping R/T dependence on drugs/alcohol, inability to manage stress, manipulative behavior	Prior to discharge: Expresses feelings regarding (specify) Identifies alternative positive coping strategies
Ineffective family coping: disabling R/T inability to accept member's dependence on drugs/alcohol	Prior to discharge, family members: Express feelings regarding dependence of member on drugs/alcohol Identify positive strategies to deal with feelings
Fear R/T effects of withdrawal process, injury by other clients, confinement, absence of drugs/alcohol	Expresses decreased fear within __ days
Powerlessness R/T perceived inability to remain drug/alcohol-free, lack of skill in managing without drugs/alcohol	Prior to discharge or within __ days: Verbalizes positive feelings about ability to control drug/alcohol use
Chronic low self-esteem R/T feelings of guilt, powerlessness	Prior to discharge: Verbalizes positive feelings about self __ times daily Identifies strengths and ability to utilize them to remain drug/alcohol-free
Sensory/perceptual alterations: visual/tactile R/T effects of intoxication, withdrawal	Prior to discharge, no evidence of visual/tactile hallucinations
Impaired social interaction R/T fear of rejection	Interacts with others at least __ times per __ (time frame)

Text continued on following page

Substance Abuse *Continued*

Nursing Diagnosis	Client Outcomes
Social isolation R/T desire to avoid hazardous peer group	Prior to discharge identifies alternative sources for social interaction
High risk for violence: self-directed or directed at others R/T effects of intoxication, withdrawal, impaired perception	During hospitalization, no evidence of injury to self or others
High risk for trauma R/T impaired judgment, effects of drug/alcohol intoxication/withdrawal	No evidence of accident or injury throughout hospitalization
High risk for aspiration R/T overdose of drugs/alcohol	No evidence of aspiration throughout hospitalization
Knowledge deficit (disease process, effects of prolonged use of drugs/alcohol, treatment options, support systems, follow-up care)	Prior to discharge, client/family: Describes addiction process Identifies the hazards associated with prolonged use of drugs/alcohol Lists three treatment options Identifies available support systems Indicates the need for and identifies personal plan for follow-up care

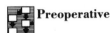 **Preoperative**

Nursing Diagnosis	Client Outcomes
Sleep pattern disturbance R/T fear of outcome of procedure, hospital environment	Experiences at least 3 uninterrupted hours of sleep twice during the night prior to surgery
Fear R/T outcome of surgery, unfamiliar environment	Verbalizes decreased fear prior to surgery
Anticipatory grieving R/T potential loss or change of body part/function	Prior to surgery, verbalizes feelings about potential changes
Knowledge deficit (surgical routine, postoperative care)	Prior to surgery, describes preoperative routines and anticipated postoperative care

Postoperative

Nursing Diagnosis	Client Outcomes
High risk for altered peripheral tissue perfusion R/T hypovolemia, hypothermia	Within 24 hours following surgery: B/P, P WNL for client Temperature WNL
Ineffective breathing pattern R/T anxiety, pain, effects of anesthesia	Respiratory rate, rhythm, and depth WNL for client within 24 hours
High risk for aspiration R/T retained secretions, effects of anesthesia, pain	No evidence of aspiration postoperatively
High risk for fluid volume deficit R/T profuse wound drainage, excessive vomiting, N/G tube drainage	Within ___ days following surgery: No evidence of excessive wound/tube drainage B/P WNL for client Balanced I&O
Altered nutrition: less than body requirements R/T anorexia, vomiting, increased nutritional needs	Following surgery, weight loss no greater than ___ lb
Pain R/T effects of tissue trauma, N/V, abdominal distention	Expresses comfort within ___ minutes after initiation of comfort measure
High risk for altered oral mucous membrane R/T mouth breathing, dehydration	Moist oral mucous membranes throughout hospitalization
High risk for altered skin integrity, R/T irritating wound drainage, immobility	No evidence of skin breakdown over bony prominences or in incisional area throughout hospitalization
Activity intolerance R/T fatigue, pain, effects of medication	B/P and P WNL for client during periods of activity
Impaired physical mobility R/T pain, effects of medication, fear of injury	Following surgery, increases mobility consistent with physical ability

Nursing Diagnosis	Client Outcomes
Self-care deficit (specify) R/T pain, activity intolerance, fear of injury	Performs ADLs within physical limitations following surgery
Urinary retention R/T flat position, anxiety, pain	Following surgery: No evidence of bladder distention Voids at least 240 ml q shift
Colonic constipation R/T effects of drugs, decreased fluid intake, decreased mobility	Resumes normal bowel patterns q ___ prior to discharge
Sleep-pattern disturbance R/T pain, hospital routine, anxiety	Experiences at least 4 hours of uninterrupted sleep twice within 24 hours
High risk for trauma R/T weakness, effects of drugs, hypotension	No evidence of accident or injury postoperatively
Fear R/T outcome of surgical procedure, pain, postoperative care	Within 36 hours after surgery, verbalizes decreased feelings of fear
Knowledge deficit (wound care, postoperative complications, diet, activity, follow-up care)	Prior to discharge, client/ family: Demonstrates correct wound care Names indications of postoperative complications and describes methods of prevention Selects high-protein foods from menu Explains activity limitations Describes the need for and identifies plans for follow-up care

Differential Diagnosis

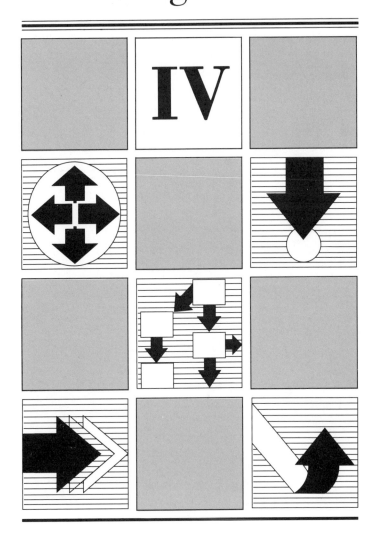

IV

Often, nurses find that many nursing diagnoses are similar to one another; therefore, during the diagnostic process it is somewhat difficult to differentiate among them. In this part of the text, 30 diagnoses are presented in a format that allows the reader to identify the similarities and differences among diagnoses that are closely related or frequently confused. For each set of diagnoses, a brief case study is presented along with the nursing diagnoses that might be considered. In addition, the definitions, common defining characteristics, and related/risk factors as well as differentiating defining characteristics and related/risk factors are presented for each set. Finally, the correct diagnosis is identified. A list of diagnoses included in this part with their corresponding page numbers is shown in the accompanying table.

Difficult-to-Differentiate Diagnoses

■ Case Study

Margaret Ross has been hospitalized for over 2 weeks in the critical care area with a diagnosis of acute respiratory failure secondary to chronic airway limitation. She is ventilator-dependent, despite attempts to wean her off the ventilator. The nursing staff have taught Margaret how to write notes to communicate her needs and how to point to pictures. She writes, "Leave me alone, I want to die. If I hadn't smoked for so many years I wouldn't be on this machine. I have no control over my breathing. I don't want to live like this."

Hopelessness or Powerlessness?

Definition

Hopelessness: The subjective state in which an individual sees limited or no alternatives or personal choices available and is unable to mobilize energy on own behalf

Powerlessness: The state in which an individual experiences the perception that one's own actions will not significantly affect an outcome or a perceived lack of control over a current situation or immediate happening

---

	Hopelessness	Powerlessness
Defining Characteristics Common to Both		
Apathy	√	√
Withdrawal	√	√
Lack of involvement in care	√	√
Depression	√	√
Defining Characteristics Differentiating		
Anger		√
Violent behavior		√
Anxiety		√

	Hopelessness	Powerlessness
Defining Characteristics Differentiating		
Resentment		√
Guilt		√
Expressions of doubt about self or role performance		√
Decreased appetite	√	
Related Factors in Common		
Social isolation	√	√
Activity restriction	√	√
Role disruption	√	√
Depression	√	√
Related Factors Differentiating		
Communication barriers		√
Grieving	√	
Lost belief in religious values	√	
Health care environment		√
Lack of knowledge or skills		√
Lifestyle of helplessness		√

Answer to Case Study: Powerlessness

■ **Case Study**

A new resident, Bill Langley, age 83, has been admitted to your long-term care facility. He is agitated, saying, "One two three hike, cross the goal line, round the bend, here he goes, what is for dinner, tra la la, on the right." He is disoriented and unable to supply any answers to your questions. You place Bill in a room with another resident and introduce him to his roommate. Bill says, "He's from the FBI, FBI, come to kill me, FBI, FBI." Bill remains obsessed with the idea that his roommate is out to get him, despite your reassurances.

Altered Thought Processes or Sensory Perceptual Alteration?

Definition

Altered Thought Processes: The state in which the individual experiences a disruption in cognitive operations and activities

Sensory/Perceptual Alterations: A state in which an individual experiences a change in the amount or patterning of oncoming stimuli accompanied by a diminished, exaggerated, distorted, or impaired response to such stimuli

---

	Altered Thought Processes	Sensory/Perceptual Alterations
Defining Characteristics Common to Both		
Hallucinations	√	√
Agitation	√	√
Depression	√	√
Disorientation to time, place, person	√	√
Bizarre thinking	√	√
Lack of concentration	√	√
Change in problem solving, abstraction abilities	√	√

	Altered Thought Processes	Sensory/Perceptual Alterations
Defining Characteristics Common to Both		
Inappropriate responses/behavior	√	√
Altered communication patterns	√	√
Defining Characteristics Differentiating		
Visual and auditory distortions		√
Motor incoordination		√
Rapid mood swings		√
Reported or necessitated change in sensory acuity		√
Obsessions	√	
Related Factors in Common		
Sleep deprivation	√	√
Side effects of medications	√	√
Psychological stress	√	√
Social isolation	√	√
Anxiety	√	√
Sensory deprivation	√	√
Related Factors Differentiating		
Inability to communicate, speak, understand, respond		√

Text continued on following page

	Altered Thought Processes	Sensory/Perceptual Alterations
Related Factors Differentiating		
Fear of the unknown	√	
Effects of aging	√	
Effects of neurological disease, trauma, or deficit		√
Altered sensory reception, transmission, and/or integration		√
Loss of memory	√	
Impaired judgment	√	

Answer to Case Study: Altered Thought Processes

■ Case Study

As you are driving down the road one morning, you come upon a car flipped over on its roof. A man is lying on the road. The police and ambulance have not yet arrived. When you kneel next to the man, your nursing assessment reveals the following information: The man is alert and oriented. He denies blacking out and says he crawled out of the car after it flipped over. His pulse is rapid and he is trembling. He keeps glancing at his car in a worried manner but does not volunteer information unless you ask him specific questions.

Anxiety or Fear?

Definition

Anxiety: The state in which an individual experiences a vague uneasy feeling, the source of which is often nonspecific or unknown.

Fear: A state in which an individual experiences feelings of dread related to an identifiable source perceived as dangerous

---

	Anxiety	Fear
Defining Characteristics Common to Both		
Crying	√	√
Sympathetic stimulation (increase in blood pressure, pulse, respirations)	√	√
Diaphoresis	√	√
Urinary frequency	√	√
Trembling	√	√
Insomnia	√	√
Increased alertness	√	√
Feelings of inadequacy	√	√
Agitated	√	√

Text continued on following page

	Anxiety	Fear
Defining Characteristics Differentiating		
Withdrawn		√
Panicked		√
Worried	√	
Terrified		√
Afraid of unspecific consequences	√	
Increased questioning/verbalization		√
Difficulty expressing self	√	
Related Factors in Common		
Loss of significant other	√	√
Threat of death	√	√
Knowledge deficit	√	√
Feelings of failure	√	√
Threat to or change in health status	√	√
Related Factors Differentiating		
Interpersonal transmission and contagion		√
Sensory impairment, deprivation, or overload		√
Unconscious conflict about essential values and goals of life	√	

Answer to Case Study: Anxiety

■ Case Study

Willard Jensen, age 62, has been referred to the community mental health center by his family practitioner who has been treating him for unresolved peptic ulcer disease for 18 months. During the initial intake interview, Willard gives the following history: Two years ago Willard's wife and son were killed in a motor vehicle accident. Eighteen months ago, Willard's only sister died from cancer. Six months ago, Willard's daughter, with whom he had been living, moved across the country when her corporation transferred her to a new office. During the assessment, you note that Willard gives short monotone answers to your questions. He has difficulty expressing his feelings about these multiple losses, saying, "Men are supposed to be tough and handle these things well." It is clear that Willard has not shaved or bathed for several days. The clothes he is wearing appear to be two sizes too big for him. Willard states that he has been missing a lot of work lately because he is unable to get out of bed and has trouble concentrating on his job when he does go to work.

Anticipatory Grieving or Dysfunctional Grieving?

Definition
Anticipatory Grieving: Grieving begins *before* the loss occurs
Dysfunctional Grieving: Grieving is an exaggerated response

	Anticipatory Grieving	Dysfunctional Grieving
Defining Characteristics Common to Both		
Guilt	√	√
Anger	√	√
Denial	√	√
Sorrow	√	√
Changes in activity levels	√	√

Text continued on following page

	Anticipatory Grieving	Dysfunctional Grieving
Defining Characteristics Common to Both		
Crying	√	√
Altered communication patterns	√	√
Defining Characteristics Differentiating		
Interference with life functioning		√
Suicidal thoughts		√
Prolonged anger and hostility		√
Exaggerated expressions of guilt for more than 12–18 months		√
Related Factors in Common		
Effects of actual or potential loss of significant other, health or social status, or valued object	√	√
Related Factors Differentiating		
Absence of anticipatory grieving		√
Thwarted grieving		√
Effects of multiple losses or crises		√
Lack of resolution of previous grieving response		√
Decreased support system		√

Answer to Case Study: Dysfunctional Grieving

■ **Case Study**

Juan Torres is a 32-year-old HIV-positive heroin addict. As the nurse practitioner at the methadone clinic, you notice that Juan is particularly agitated today. He is pacing around the waiting area, saying, ''He's telling me I have to shoot myself. I'm a bad person. He's looking at my woman and I deserve to lose her.'' When you ask Juan questions, he becomes more upset, and repeats his statements about wanting to shoot himself.

High Risk for Violence or High Risk for Self-Mutilation?

Definition

High Risk for Violence: Self-Directed or Directed at Others: The state in which an individual experiences a predisposition to violent, destructive acts directed toward self or others

High Risk for Self-Mutilation: A state in which an individual is at high risk to perform a deliberate act upon the self with the intent to injure, not kill, which produces immediate tissue damage to the body

---

	High Risk for Violence: Self-Directed or Directed at Others	High Risk for Self-Mutilation
Defining Characteristics Common to Both: None (As a high-risk diagnosis, they have no defining characteristics)		
Risk Factors in Common		
Clients with borderline personality disorders/ manipulative/antisocial	√	√
Clients in psychotic states	√	√
Emotionally disturbed and/or battered children	√	√
Clients with a history of self-injury	√	√

Text continued on following page

	High Risk for Violence: Self-Directed or Directed at Others	**High Risk for Self-Mutilation**
Defining Characteristics Common to Both: None (As a high-risk diagnosis, they have no defining characteristics)		
Risk Factors in Common		
Command hallucinations	√	√
Depression	√	√
Feelings of rejection	√	√
Risk Factors Differentiating		
Toxic reaction to medications	√	
Substance abuse or withdrawal	√	
Significant change in lifestyle	√	

Answer to Case Study: High Risk for Violence: Self-Directed

■ Case Study

Thelma Rowens is a 50-year-old woman with asthma. She has been hospitalized every 6 months when her symptoms worsen. As the case manager for clients with pulmonary disorders, you have noticed this pattern of frequent hospitalizations. When you enter Thelma's hospital room you smell cigarette smoke seeping out from under the bathroom door. In the process of talking with Thelma, you obtain the following information: Despite education, Thelma has continued to allow her cat to sleep on her bed. She says, "I'm sure that my cat has nothing to do with my lungs. Also, a few cigarettes a day can't hurt."

Noncompliance or Ineffective Management of Therapeutic Regimen?

Definition

Noncompliance: The state in which an individual is unwilling or unable to adhere to a therapeutic recommendation

Ineffective Management of Therapeutic Regimen: A pattern of regulating and integrating into daily living a program for treatment of illness and the sequelae of illness that is unsatisfactory for meeting specific health goals

---

	Noncompliance	Ineffective Management of Therapeutic Regimen
Defining Characteristics Common to Both		
Acceleration of illness symptoms	√	√
Nonadherence to therapeutic regimen	√	√
Making inappropriate choices of daily living for meeting goals of a treatment or prevention program	√	√

Text continued on following page

	Noncompliance	Ineffective Management of Therapeutic Regimen
Defining Characteristics Differentiating		
Verbalized desire to manage the treatment of illness and prevention of sequelae		√
Failure to seek care when disease status warrants	√	
Failure to keep appointments	√	
Nonadherence after education	√	
Verbalized difficulty with regulation/integration of one or more prescribed regimens for treatment of illness and its effects or prevention of complications		√
Related Factors in Common		
Complexity of therapeutic regimen	√	√
Relationship between client and provider	√	√
Economic difficulties	√	√
Lack of support system	√	√
Knowledge deficit	√	√
Perceived benefits of regimen	√	√
Powerlessness	√	√
Cultural values	√	√
Related Factors Differentiating		
Side effects of medications	√	

	Noncompliance	Ineffective Management of Therapeutic Regimen
Related Factors Differentiating		
Impaired ability to perform tasks	√	
Denial	√	
Depression	√	
Forgetfulness	√	
Decisional conflicts		√
Family conflicts		√

Answer to Case Study: Noncompliance

■ Case Study

Susan Young is a 27-year-old woman who has been married for less than 2 years. Because of a positive family history for breast cancer and diagnosed fibrocystic disease, she has routinely had mammograms since age 21. Her last study was positive for a 4-mm mass for which she elected to have a radical mastectomy. When she returns for her postoperative check-up, she bursts into tears when the office nurse asks her how she feels. "I feel so ugly—I wouldn't blame Keith if he never wanted to look at me again. This scar is so ugly that I don't even want him to see or touch me. All I do is think about how ugly I look and how much I would give to have my breast back."

Body Image Disturbance or Self-Esteem Disturbance?

Definition

Body Image Disturbance: The state in which an individual experiences a negative or distorted perception of the body

Self-Esteem Disturbance: The state in which an individual has negative self-evaluation/feelings about self or capabilities, which may be directly or indirectly expressed

	Body Image Disturbance	Self-Esteem Disturbance
Defining Characteristics Common to Both		
Negative verbal response	√	√
Negative nonverbal response	√	√
Defining Characteristics Differentiating		
Verbalizes fear of or rejection by others	√	
Self-negating verbalization		√
Emphasis on remaining strengths, heightened achievement	√	

	Body Image Disturbance	Self-Esteem Disturbance
Defining Characteristics Differentiating		
Rationalizes/rejects positive feedback and exaggerates negative feedback about self		√
Denies problems obvious to others		√
Preoccupied with change or loss of body part/function	√	
Related Factors in Common		(Self-Esteem Disturbance has no identified related factors)

Answer to case study: Body Image Disturbance

■ **Case Study**

Baby Sims is a 3-week-old premature infant of 32 weeks' gestation who weighed 1675 g at birth. The neonatal nursery nurse, in explaining his condition to his young parents, tells them that his skin color changes from pink to blue frequently, that his heart rate and respirations fluctuate between very high and low rates. She also tells them that although his temperature is elevated at this time, it often fluctuates from very low to very high levels. These changes are particularly significant when the baby is moved from the isolette or when he is bathed.

Hyperthermia or Ineffective Thermoregulation?

Definition

Hyperthermia: The state in which an individual is at risk because the body temperature is elevated above the individual's normal range

Ineffective Thermoregulation: The state in which an individual's temperature fluctuates between hypothermia and hyperthermia

---

	Hyperthermia	Ineffective Thermoregulation
Defining Characteristics Common to Both		
Changes in skin color	√	√
Changes in skin temperature	√	√
Changes in heart rate	√	√
Changes in respiratory rate	√	√
Defining Characteristics Differentiating		
Increased body temperature	√	
Fluctuating body temperature		√
Related Factors in Common		
Effects of trauma/illness	√	√

	Hyperthermia	Ineffective Thermoregulation
Related Factors in Common		
Effects of medication	√	√
Effects of aging	√	√
Inappropriate clothing	√	√
Related Factors Differentiating		
Effects of immaturity		√
Fluctuating environmental temperature		√
Exposure to hot environment	√	
Dehydration	√	
Increased metabolic rate	√	

Answer to Case Study: Ineffective Thermoregulation

■ **Case Study**

Tim O'Donovan is a 14-year-old second-semester college freshman at a prestigious Ivy League University. He was referred to the nurse practitioner at the College Health Service by his counselor. In talking to Tim, the nurse determines that he is feeling rejected by his peers, angry, and very alone in the college community. He says he is uncomfortable in most group situations and is unable to identify individuals or groups that might be of assistance to him. Tim's last comment to the nurse is "Doogie Howser on TV makes it look like this should be easy, but I feel like no one likes me and they just don't want me around because we have nothing in common!"

Impaired Social Interaction or Social Isolation?

Definition

Impaired Social Interaction: The state in which an individual participates in an insufficient or excessive quantity or ineffective quality of social exchange

Social Isolation: Aloneness experienced by the individual and perceived as imposed by others and as a negative or threatened state

---

	Impaired Social Interaction	Social Isolation
Defining Characteristics Common to Both		
Verbalized or observed discomfort in social situations	√	√
Defining Characteristics Differentiating		
Use of unsuccessful social behaviors	√	
Dysfunctional interaction with peers, family, and/or others	√	

	Impaired Social Interaction	Social Isolation
Defining Characteristics Differentiating		
Expresses feelings of aloneness imposed by others		√
Expresses feelings of rejection		√
Related Factors in Common		
Inadequate support systems/ personal resources	√	√
Sociocultural dissonance	√	√
Related Factors Differentiating		
Lack of knowledge/ skills to enhance socialization	√	
Communication barriers	√	
Therapeutic isolation	√	
Environmental barriers		√
Altered mental status, physical appearance, state of wellness		√
Delay in accomplishing developmental tasks		√

Answer to Case Study: Social Isolation

■ Case Study

Frank Barnaby is a 36-year-old black male who needs a coronary artery bypass graft after a recent myocardial infarction. The nurse observes the interaction between Frank and his spouse following a meeting when the physician tells them that he needs the surgery immediately based on the results of his cardiac catheterization. Frank's wife Marie is crying and says, "You'll never make it through the surgery and all the changes afterward." Frank replies, "I'm just going to have to do whatever it takes to get well." Marie continues, "You've got to be kidding—why, if I wasn't there to do all the right things for you, you wouldn't have made it through the heart attack." Frank replies, "I think I can do this." But Marie continues, "You don't listen, you don't eat the right things, and we'll never get through this." This pattern continues throughout their conversation until Frank says, "Well, do you think I should forget about the surgery then?" Marie tells him that he'll have to make up his own mind, but she doesn't see how they can do this and it can't be that bad—after all, he is so young. The next day Frank tells the nurse that he is not going to have the surgery.

Ineffective Family Coping: Compromised or Disabling?

Definition

Ineffective Family Coping: Compromised: A usually supportive primary person (family member or close friend) is providing insufficient, ineffective, or compromised support, comfort, assistance, or encouragement, which may be needed by the client to manage or master adaptive tasks related to his or her health challenge

Ineffective Family Coping: Disabling: Behavior of significant person (family member or other primary person) that disables his or her own capacities and the client's capacities to address effectively tasks essential to either person's adaptation to the health challenge

---

	Ineffective Family Coping: Compromised	Ineffective Family Coping: Disabling
Defining Characteristics Common to Both		
Excessive vigilance/ overprotection of family member	√	√
Exploitation, neglect, or withdrawal from family member	√	√
Defining Characteristics Differentiating		
Ineffective responses to illness, disability, or situational crises	√	
Expressed concern about significant other's response to health problem	√	
Denial of existence or severity of illness of family member		√
Inability to demonstrate supportive behaviors	√	
Impaired intimacy or closeness	√	
Despair, rejection, or desertion		√
Child, spousal, or elder abuse		√
Related Factors in Common		
Lack of support for family members	√	√
Effects of illness/ death of family member	√	√

Text continued on following page

	Ineffective Family Coping: Compromised	Ineffective Family Coping: Disabling
Related Factors Differentiating		
Temporary family disorganization and role changes	√	
Highly ambivalent family relationships/ marital discord		√
Isolation of family members from one another	√	
Chronically unexpressed feelings of guilt, despair, anxiety, or hostility		√
Unrealistic expectations	√	

Answer to Case Study: Ineffective Family Coping: Disabling

■ Case Study

Roberta Sedia is a 60-year-old woman referred to an outpatient pain clinic. During the interview, she reports that one night approximately 1 year ago, she awakened and was unable to move or feel her lower extremities. Her physician diagnosed her condition as transverse myelitis, an infection of the spinal cord. After 3 months of hospitalization and rehabilitation, she regained movement and feeling in both lower extremities but has persistent back pain radiating to her right thigh. She admits that over the past 6 months, she has been unable to resume her normal activities, has gained weight, and has periods when she cries for no reason at all. She verbalizes that she thinks everything would be OK if she could just get rid of the pain.

Pain or Chronic Pain?

> **Definition**
> *Pain:* A state in which an individual experiences and reports the presence of severe discomfort or an uncomfortable sensation
> *Chronic Pain:* A state in which an individual experiences pain that continues for more than 6 months

	Pain	Chronic Pain
Defining Characteristics Common to Both		
Verbal reports of pain	√	√
Facial mask of pain	√	√
Physical and social withdrawal	√	√
Guarded movement	√	√
Defining Characteristics Differentiating		
Duration of pain longer than 6 months		√

Text continued on following page

	Pain	Chronic Pain
Defining Characteristics Differentiating		
Autonomic responses to pain (vital signs, diaphoresis)	✓	
Personality changes		✓
Weight changes		✓
Clutching of painful area	✓	
Related Factors in Common		
Inflammation	✓	✓
Muscle spasm	✓	✓
Related Factors Differentiating		
Effects of surgery/ trauma	✓	
Experienced during diagnostic procedures	✓	
Overactivity	✓	
Immobility	✓	
Effects of chronic or terminal illness		✓
Chronic psychosocial disability		✓

Answer to Case Study: Chronic Pain

■ Case Study

Dean Marks is a 28-year-old computer programmer who recently lost his job in Silicon Valley. He was referred to the clinical nurse specialist in the mental health clinic by his primary care physician, who had been following him for a variety of somatic complaints. He relates to the nurse that he lost his job 6 months ago and believes that the layoff was all his fault. He believes that if he was more skilled at his job, it would not have happened. Dean also reports that he is embarrassed by the fact that he has worked for 6 different companies in the last 5 years and indicates that he was "let go" for a variety of nebulous reasons. He feels that he is "stuck in a rut" and cannot face the process of having to find another job. The nurse notes that Dean avoided eye contact throughout the interview.

Chronic Low Self-Esteem or Situational Low Self-Esteem?

Definition

Chronic Low Self-Esteem: Long standing negative self evaluation/ feelings about self or self capabilities.

Situational Low Self-Esteem: Negative self evaluation/feelings about self which develop in response to a loss or change in an individual who previously had a positive self evaluation.

	Chronic Low Self-Esteem	Situational Low Self-Esteem
Defining Characteristics Common to Both		
Expressions of guilt or shame	√	√
Indecisive	√	√
Self-negating verbalizations	√	√
Evaluates self as unable to handle situations/events	√	√
Defining Characteristics Differentiating		
Symptoms are long-standing	√	

Text continued on following page

	Chronic Low Self-Esteem	Situational Low Self-Esteem
Defining Characteristics Differentiating		
Episodic occurrence of negative self-appraisal		√
Frequent lack of success in work or other life events	√	
Seeks reassurance excessively	√	
Related Factors in Common	(No related factors have been identified for these diagnoses)	

Answer to Case Study: Chronic Low Self-Esteem

■ Case Study

Michelle Shiano is a 32-year-old mother of twins. During the delivery process, her uterus ruptured and an emergency hysterectomy was performed. Two days postoperatively, Michelle developed signs and symptoms of an infection and required third-generation antibiotics. Her pediatrician advised her that breastfeeding while on antibiotics was not recommended. The lactation specialist was consulted, who agreed with the pediatrician's recommendation. Michelle expressed her disappointment and expressed her desire to continue breastfeeding.

Ineffective Breastfeeding, Interrupted Breastfeeding, or Ineffective Infant Feeding Pattern?

Definition

Ineffective Breastfeeding: The state in which a mother, infant, or child experiences dissatisfaction or difficulty with the breastfeeding process

Interrupted Breastfeeding: A break in the continuity of the breastfeeding process as a result of inability or inadvisability of putting baby to breast for feeding

Ineffective Infant Feeding Pattern: A state in which an infant demonstrates an impaired ability to suck or coordinate the suck-swallow response

---

	Ineffective Breastfeeding	Interrupted Breastfeeding	Ineffective Infant Feeding Pattern
Defining Characteristics in Common			
Insufficient opportunity for sucking at the breast	√	√	√

Text continued on following page

	Ineffective Breastfeeding	Interrupted Breastfeeding	Ineffective Infant Feeding Pattern
Defining Characteristics Differentiating			
Verbalization of unsatisfactory breastfeeding process	√		
Infant does not receive nourishment at breast for some or all of feedings		√	
Actual or perceived inadequate milk supply	√		
Inability to initiate or sustain an effective suck			√
Inability to coordinate sucking, swallowing, and breathing			√
Maternal desire to maintain lactation and provide her breast milk for her infant's nutritional needs		√	
Related Factors in Common			
Prematurity	√	√	√

	Ineffective Breastfeeding	Interrupted Breastfeeding	Ineffective Infant Feeding Pattern
Related Factors Differentiating			
Previous history of breastfeeding failure	√		
Maternal or infant illness		√	
Maternal employment		√	
Neurological impairment/delay			√

Answer to Case Study: Interrupted Breastfeeding

■ Case Study

Kelley Morris is a 26-year-old who had a thoracotomy for a cardiac injury secondary to multiple trauma. On the second postoperative day, even though her lung has completely re-expanded, the nurse notes that there are decreased breath sounds on the affected side, elevated temperature, and rapid/shallow respirations. Kelly does not cough effectively and says that she is tired and that it hurts too much when she tries. Deep endotracheal suctioning is productive of thick mucus.

Impaired Gas Exchange, Ineffective Airway Clearance, or Ineffective Breathing Pattern?

> **Definition**
>
> **Impaired Gas Exchange:** The state in which an individual experiences a decreased passage of oxygen and/or carbon dioxide between the alveoli of the lungs and the vascular system
>
> **Ineffective Airway Clearance:** The state in which an individual is unable to clear secretions or obstructions from the respiratory tract to maintain airway patency
>
> **Ineffective Breathing Pattern:** The state in which an individual's inhalation or exhalation pattern does not enable adequate pulmonary inflation or emptying

	Impaired Gas Exchange	Ineffective Airway Clearance	Ineffective Breathing Pattern
Defining Characteristics in Common			
Cyanosis	√	√	√
Tachycardia	√	√	
Restlessness	√	√	
Cough		√	√
Abnormal blood gases	√		√
Changes in respiratory rate/depth		√	√

	Impaired Gas Exchange	Ineffective Airway Clearance	Ineffective Breathing Pattern
Defining Characteristics Differentiating			
Hypoxia	√		
Ineffective cough		√	
Pursed lip breathing and prolonged expiratory phase			√
Assumption of 3-point position			√
Related Factors in Common			
Effects of anesthesia/ medication	√	√	√
Inhalation of toxic fumes/substances	√	√	
Decreased energy, fatigue		√	√
Related Factors Differentiating			
Altered blood flow, oxygen-carrying capacity of blood, oxygen supply	√		
Alveolar capillary membrane changes	√		
Tracheobronchial secretions or obstruction		√	

Text continued on following page

	Impaired Gas Exchange	Ineffective Airway Clearance	Ineffective Breathing Pattern
Related Factors Differentiating			
Aspiration of foreign matter		√	
Cognitive, musculoskeletal, neuromuscular impairment			√
Pain/discomfort			√

Answer to Case Study: Ineffective Airway Clearance

■ Index

Note: Page numbers followed by f refer to figures; those followed by t refer to tables.

Notes

Notes